Wound Healing for Plastic Surgeons

Guest Editor

MARK S. GRANICK, MD

CLINICS IN PLASTIC SURGERY

www.plasticsurgery.theclinics.com

July 2012 • Volume 39 • Number 3

SAUNDERS an imprint of ELSEVIER, Inc.

W.B. SAUNDERS COMPANY
A Division of Elsevier Inc.

1600 John F. Kennedy Boulevard ● Suite 1800 ● Philadelphia, Pennsylvania 19103-2899

http://www.theclinics.com

CLINICS IN PLASTIC SURGERY Volume 39, Number 3
July 2012 ISSN 0094-1298, ISBN-13: 978-1-4557-4926-3

Editor: Joanne Husovski

Clinics in Plastic Surgery (ISSN 0094-1298) is published quarterly by Elsevier Inc., 360 Park Avenue South, New York, NY 10010-1710. Months of issue are January, April, July, and October. Business and Editorial Offices: 1600 John F. Kennedy Blvd., Suite 1800, Philadelphia, PA 19103-2899. Periodicals postage paid at New York, NY and additional mailing offices. Subscription prices are $448.00 per year for US individuals, $666.00 per year for US institutions, $221.00 per year for US students and residents, $509.00 per year for Canadian individuals, $779.00 per year for Canadian institutions, $578.00 per year for international individuals, $779.00 per year for international institutions, and $279.00 per year for Canadian and foreign students/residents. To receive student/resident rate, orders must be accompanied by name of affiliated institution, date of term, and the *signature* of program/residency coordinator on institution letterhead. Orders will be billed at individual rate until proof of status is received. Foreign air speed delivery is included in all *Clinics* subscription prices. All prices are subject to change without notice. **POSTMASTER:** Send address changes to *Clinics in Plastic Surgery*, Elsevier Health Sciences Division, Subscription Customer Service, 3251 Riverport Lane, Maryland Heights, MO 63043. **Customer Service: 1-800-654-2452 (US and Canada). From outside of the United States and Canada, call 314-447-8871. Fax: 314-447-8029. E-mail: JournalsCustomerService-usa@elsevier.com (for print support); JournalsOnlineSupport-usa@ elsevier.com (for online support).**

Reprints. For copies of 100 or more of articles in this publication, please contact the Commercial Reprints Department, Elsevier Inc., 360 Park Avenue South, New York, New York 10010-1710. Tel.: (+1) 212-633-3812; Fax: (+1) 212-462-1935; E-mail: reprints@elsevier.com.

Clinics in Plastic Surgery is covered in *Current Contents, EMBASE/Excerpta Medica, Science Citation Index, MEDLINE/ PubMed (Index Medicus), ASCA,* and *ISI/BIOMED.*

Printed and bound by CPI Group (UK) Ltd, Croydon, CR0 4YY

Transferred to Digital Print 2012

Contributors

GUEST EDITOR

MARK S. GRANICK, MD, FACS
Professor of Surgery, Chief of Plastic Surgery,
New Jersey Medical School, University
of Medicine and Dentistry of New Jersey,
Newark, New Jersey

AUTHORS

KOZO AKINO, MD, PhD
Visiting Professor, Department of Plastic and
Reconstructive Surgery, Nagasaki, Japan

SADANORI AKITA, MD, PhD
Associate Professor, Department of Plastic
and Reconstructive Surgery, Nagasaki, Japan

KUNJ K. DESAI, MD
Department of Surgery, New Jersey Medical
School, University of Medicine and Dentistry
of New Jersey, Newark, New Jersey

DAVID E. EISENBUD, MD
Managing Partner, Millburn Surgical
Associates, Millburn, New Jersey

ELOF ERIKSSON, MD, PhD
Division of Plastic Surgery, Brigham and
Women's Hospital, Harvard Medical School,
Boston, Massachusetts

MARK S. GRANICK, MD, FACS
Professor of Surgery, Chief of Plastic Surgery,
New Jersey Medical School, University of
Medicine and Dentistry of New Jersey,
Newark, New Jersey

LUKE G. GUTWEIN, MD
Division of Plastic and Reconstructive Surgery,
Department of Surgery, University of Florida,
Gainesville, Florida

EDWARD HAHN, MD
Division of Plastic Surgery, Department
of Surgery, New Jersey Medical School,
University of Medicine and Dentistry of
New Jersey, Newark, New Jersey

KENJI HAYASHIDA, MD, PhD
Lecturer, Department of Plastic and
Reconstructive Surgery, Nagasaki, Japan

AKIYOSHI HIRANO, MD
Professor, Department of Plastic and
Reconstructive Surgery, Nagasaki, Japan

JOON PIO HONG, MD, PhD, MMM
Associate Professor, Department of Plastic
Surgery, Asan Medical Center, University of
Ulsan College of Medicine, Seoul, Korea

IAN C. HOPPE, MD
Division of Plastic Surgery, Department of
Surgery, New Jersey Medical School,
University of Medicine and Dentistry of New
Jersey, Newark, New Jersey

JOHAN JUNKER, PhD
Division of Plastic Surgery, Brigham and
Women's Hospital, Harvard Medical School,
Boston, Massachusetts

ELIZABETH KIWANUKA, MD
Division of Plastic Surgery, Brigham and
Women's Hospital, Harvard Medical School,
Boston, Massachusetts

EDWARD LEE, MD
Residency Program Director, Division of Plastic Surgery, New Jersey Medical School, University of Medicine and Dentistry of New Jersey, Newark, New Jersey

BRUCE A. MAST, MD
Associate Professor and Chief, Division of Plastic and Reconstructive Surgery, Department of Surgery, University of Florida, Gainesville, Florida

GIOVANNI MOSTI, MD
Head, Angiology Department, Clinica MD Barbantini, Lucca, Italy

GERIT MULDER, DPM, MS, PhD, FRCST, MAPWCA
Professor of Surgery and Orthopedics, Division of Trauma, Department of Surgery; Director, Wound Treatment and Research Center, University of California, San Diego, San Diego, California

TAE SUK OH, MD
Department of Plastic Surgery, Asan Medical Center, University of Ulsan College of Medicine, Seoul, Korea

AKIRA OHTSURU, MD, PhD
Takashi Nagai Memorial International Hibakusha Medical Center, Nagasaki University Hospital; Professor, Department of Radiation Health Management, Fukushima Medical University, Fukushima, Japan

MOUSUMEE PANIGRAHI, BS
Division of Plastic and Reconstructive Surgery, Department of Surgery, University of Florida, Gainesville, Florida

JULIAN J. PRIBAZ, MD
Professor, Division of Plastic Surgery, Department of Surgery, Brigham and Women's Hospital, Boston, Massachusetts

BENSON PULIKKOTILL, MD
Department of Surgery, New Jersey Medical School, University of Medicine and Dentistry of New Jersey, Newark, New Jersey

GREGORY S. SCHULTZ, PhD
Professor, UF Research Foundation, Department of Obstetrics and Gynecology, Institute for Wound Research, University of Florida, Gainesville, Florida

KEIJI SUZUKI, PhD
Associate Professor, Atomic Bomb Disease Institute, Nagasaki University School of Medicine, Nagasaki, Japan

SIMON G. TALBOT, MD
Instructor, Division of Plastic Surgery, Department of Surgery, Brigham and Women's Hospital, Boston, Massachusetts

MAYER TENENHAUS, MD, FACS
Professor, Plastic and Reconstructive Surgery, Department of Surgery, Division of Plastic Surgery, University of California at San Diego Medical Center, San Diego, California

KELLY WALLIN, DPM
2nd Year Podiatric Surgery Resident, Mercy Medical Center, San Diego, San Diego, California

SHUNICHI YAMASHITA, MD, PhD
Takashi Nagai Memorial International Hibakusha Medical Center, Nagasaki University Hospital; Atomic Bomb Disease Institute, Nagasaki University School of Medicine; Professor and Vice Rector, Fukushima Medical University, Fukushima, Japan

HIROSHI YOSHIMOTO, MD, PhD
Assistant Professor, Department of Plastic and Reconstructive Surgery, Nagasaki, Japan

Contents

Randomized controlled studies reveal that surgery and compression have similar effectiveness in healing ulcers but surgery is more effective in preventing recurrence. Most leg ulcers have a venous pathophysiology and occur because of venous ambulatory hypertension caused by venous reflux and impairment of the venous pumping function. Proposed surgical interventions range from crossectomy and stripping to perforator vein interruption and endovascular procedures (laser, radiofrequency). More conservative procedures (foam sclerotherapy, conservative hemodynamic treatment) have also been proposed.

This review provides a thorough and clear discussion on the outcomes of stem cells in treating chronic wounds. With recent technological developments that now allow isolation and culture of stem cells, researchers are able to perform vigorous studies on somatic or adult stem cells. Human and animal stem cell studies are discussed with a focus on the basic process of stem cells in wound healing and the authors' first-hand clinical experience with stem cells used for chronic wound healing.

Disturbances to healing observed under hypoxic conditions have given insights into the roles of oxygen. Wound hypoxia is more prevalent than generally appreciated, and occurs even in patients who are free of arterial occlusive disease. There is a strong scientific basis for oxygen treatment as prophylaxis against infection, to facilitate wound closure, and to prevent amputation in wounded patients. This article reviews extensive data from preclinical and human trials of supplemental inhaled oxygen, hyperbaric oxygen, and topical oxygen treatment. Oxygen supports biochemical metabolism and cellular function, and has roles in combating infection and facilitating the wound healing cascade.

Negative pressure wound therapy (NPWT) has overwhelmed the wound-healing world. A systematic review puts it into perspective. The authors have developed an algorithm after careful evaluation and analysis of the scientific literature supporting the use of these devices. This article describes mechanisms of action, technical considerations, wound preparation, and clinical evidence, reviews the literature, and discusses NPWT use in specific wounds, such as diabetic foot ulcers, open abdomen, pressure ulcers, open fractures, sterna wounds, grafts, and flaps. Contraindications for and complications of NPWT are outlined, and specific recommendations given for the situations in which the authors use NPWT.

This article is a discussion and presentation for plastic surgeons, in which each section is dedicated to a principle necessary for complex wound reconstruction. Each principle is discussed and includes detailed images of the associated operations.

CLINICS IN PLASTIC SURGERY

Plastic Surgery's Critical Role in Wound Management

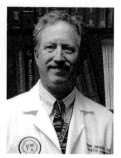

Mark S. Granick, MD
Guest Editor

I have edited a number of issues of *Clinics in Plastic Surgery* relating to wound issues: 1993 Management of Radiation Wounds, 1998 Wound Healing: State of the Art, and Wound Surgery in 2007. The evolving theme of this series of wound editions is to maintain Plastic Surgery's pre-eminence in the field of surgical wound management. The past two decades have been a time of intense technologic development with regard to wound management. Since there are so many exciting advances in wound technology, it is critical for all plastic surgeons to be up-to-date on this topic. Wound technology has enabled us to treat a wide variety of wounds successfully and has transformed wound surgery from a rather unexciting specialty to a cutting-edge specialty.

During the past decade I have had an opportunity to work with plastic surgeons throughout the world and have been part of an international team training surgeons throughout the world in wound technology. Many of the international surgeons have access to technologic advances prior to the introduction of these developments in the United States. I have assembled a group of authors for this edition who have international reputations for harnessing exciting new technologies.

The first article discusses the impact of evidence-based medicine (EBM) on the interpretation of data in the wound discipline. Debridement is a funda-mental technique for wound surgery, yet solid EBM is somewhat lacking. The article on microbial barrier protection addresses the hot topic areas of biofilm management and the use of new antimicrobial agents and dressings. Clinical use of growth factors in modulating wound response is another area of exciting translational research reviewed in article 3 by the leaders of this field. Regenerative materials are now an everyday item for the wound surgeon, yet many surgeons are not familiar with the spectrum of available technologies and how to incorporate them into practical use. Venous leg ulcers continue to plague millions of people, but the pathway to improvement lies in the proper use of available techniques as well as the incorporation of new technologies. Stem cells are an exciting area of wound research and the earliest data on the clinical use of stem cells is coming out of Japan. Hyperbaric oxygen (HBO) is a technology that has been around for years, but due to poor initial research, overuse, and abuse, it has been largely misunderstood. Article 7 integrates the proper use of HBO into the comprehensive surgical care of the wound patient. Negative pressure wound therapy (NPWT) has seen the growth of industrial competitors in the last few years. It is a widely used technique. Article 8 discusses the use and application of NPWT to maximize efficacy and reduce cost. The final two articles deal with the amazing results that

plasticsurgery.theclinics.com

Clin Plastic Surg 39 (2012) ix–x
doi:10.1016/j.cps.2012.05.005

specialized plastic surgical teams can accomplish using very sophisticated surgical technique and technology.

My hope is that this publication will further solidify the critical role of Plastic Surgery in wound management. I also hope to encourage plastic surgeons throughout the world to continue their excellent work in this important area of medicine and surgery.

Mark S. Granick, MD
Division of Plastic Surgery
New Jersey Medical School-UMDNJ
140 Bergen Street E1620
Newark, NJ 07103, USA

E-mail address:
mgranickmd@umdnj.edu

Debridement of Chronic Wounds
A Qualitative Systematic Review of Randomized Controlled Trials

Ian C. Hoppe, MD, Mark S. Granick, MD*

KEYWORDS

- Debridement • Wound healing • Chronic wounds

KEY POINTS

- Routine use of debridement in the treatment of acute and chronic wounds became surgical dogma because it represented a life saving advance in wound management.
- Debridement in the management of acute and chronic wounds is a fairly recent development in the history of surgery.
- The evolution of debridement is not necessarily supported by evidence-based medicine because of the difficulty in performing randomized controlled trials due to ethical concerns.

INTRODUCTION

The routine use of debridement in the management of acute and chronic wounds represents a life-saving advancement in wound management and is a fairly recent development in the history of surgery. The evolution of debridement is not necessarily supported by evidence-based medicine because of the drastic improvement in patient survival after its adoption.

Theories of Wound Management

Hippocrates advocated keeping wounds dry, whereas Galen proposed the theory of laudable pus.[1,2] This latter theory, which advocated the practice of encouraging wounds to suppurate, was adopted by much of ancient civilization because of Galen's prolific writing on the subject. Therefore, very little progress was made in wound management until the 14th century. The next 4 centuries saw the adoption of surgery by barbers, with limited advancements in the treatment of wounds.[3,4] The term debridement was introduced

by Pierre Joseph Desault in the late 1700s to refer to the freshening of edges of war wounds.[2] He noted a marked increase in survival after use of this technique.

The practice of debridement progressed sporadically through the 20th century. The World Wars and other conflicts presented war surgeons with injuries inflicted by higher-energy weapon. Military surgeons again showed improved survival and limb salvage with debridement. The advent of antibiotics also allowed for increased survival in patients with wounds, and a commensurate increase in demand for the management of these patients. Debridement has subsequently become ingrained as a surgical standard of care.

Strides made in the treatment of chronic diseases, such as diabetes and venous insufficiency, have similarly increased the number of wounds that require management. A landmark study published in 1967 determined the bacterial load of a wound at which a skin graft would likely fail.[5] Various debridement techniques were subsequently shown to decrease bacterial burden.[6] More

Division of Plastic Surgery, New Jersey Medical School-UMDNJ, 140 Bergen Street E1620, Newark, NJ 07103, USA
* Corresponding author.
E-mail address: mgranickmd@umdnj.edu

Clin Plastic Surg 39 (2012) 221–228
doi:10.1016/j.cps.2012.04.001
0094-1298/12/$ – see front matter © 2012 Elsevier Inc. All rights reserved.

recently, entire volumes have been devoted to wound management and debridement.[7–11] Technologic advances spurred a surgical discussion of the nature of debridement and an understanding of when debridement is adequate.

Wound Bed Preparation

The introduction of expensive advanced wound therapies led to a concerted effort in the wound industry to optimize their efficacy. A meeting of medical wound-healing experts was convened in 2002 to develop a systematic approach to wound bed preparation.[12] Their consensus document advocated removing barriers to healing in preparing an appropriate wound bed before making further attempts at wound closure. These barriers include tissue necrosis, bacterial overload, moisture imbalance, and impairment of the healing tissue edge. Debridement is the most efficient and effective technique of achieving wound bed preparation. Unfortunately, the medical literature is still sparse, with high-quality studies examining the efficacy of debridement and the specific techniques. Organizing a multicenter randomized controlled trial examining the benefits of debridement compared with no treatment would essentially represent a step backward in the management of wounds because of the clinically proven benefit of debridement. In addition, the organization of this study would raise ethical concerns regarding withholding of care.

METHODS

One author (I.C.H) conducted all initial searches. Medline was searched from 1946 to July 2011 using the following Boolean search string: *debridement* (MeSH Terms) AND *randomized controlled trial* (Publication Type).

Daily updates of new papers that matched the search criteria were provided via e-mail. Titles and abstracts were screened for suitability using the following inclusion criteria:

- Clinical human study
- Wounds located externally or cutaneously
- Wounds described as chronic in nature.

One or more methods of debridement were examined. Full-text articles were retrieved and submitted to the following exclusion criteria:

- Wounds caused by burn or acute trauma
- Study did not examine an accepted method of debridement
- Unclear study design.

In addition, the Cochrane Library was searched for comprehensive reviews regarding each methodology, and these were subsequently included in each section.

RESULTS OF STUDIES

Nineteen studies were found that satisfied the inclusion and exclusion criteria (**Table 1**).

EVIDENCE FOR DEBRIDEMENT
Surgical Debridement

Although numerous forms of debridement exist, surgical debridement (**Fig. 1**) is the standard against which they are judged. Surgical debridement

- Allows direct removal of all devitalized tissue
- Allows reduction of bacterial burden
- Allows removal of desiccated tissues
- Provides the quickest method of preparing a wound bed for eventual healing
- Has become the standard of care.

A problem arises when seeking high-quality studies examining the efficacy of surgical debridement versus other methods of debridement. No randomized controlled studies exist. The reason for this is the general consensus regarding debridement and its efficacy; ethical concerns would be raised if a control group was not provided with the standard of care. An exception to this is tangential hydrosurgery.

Two studies were included that met the inclusion and exclusion criteria. A retrospective review published in 2009 of a multicenter randomized controlled trial provides perhaps the best evidence for the efficacy of surgical debridement.[13] The original randomized controlled trial examined was the phase III testing of a bioengineered dermal substitute in the treatment of venous leg ulcers and diabetic foot ulcers. The protocol for this trial included debridement to be performed at each visit if clinically indicated. Results showed that greater rates of wound closure occurred at centers at which debridement was performed more frequently.

Another intriguing multicenter randomized controlled study, published in 1996, examined the effect of recombinant human platelet-derived growth factor on the healing of diabetic foot ulcers.[14] During the course of this study, results showed that lower rates of healing occurred at centers that performed less frequent debridement.

Although these studies provide evidence that debridement is effective in managing venous leg ulcers and diabetic foot ulcers, each study experienced a difference based on centers involved in

Table 1
Characteristics of included studies

	Author(s)	Year	Study Design	Number of Wounds	Intervention
Surgical	Caputo et al[15]	2008	RCT	41	Hydrosurgery debridement vs conventional surgical debridement in lower extremity ulcers
	Cardinal et al[13]	2009	RCT; retrospective review of data	676	Comparison of rates of surgical debridement in venous leg ulcers and diabetic foot ulcers
	Steed et al[14]	1996	RCT; double-blind	118	Comparison of rates of surgical debridement in diabetic foot ulcers
Biologic	Dumville et al[18,19]	2009	RCT	267	Larval therapy vs hydrogel dressing in venous leg ulcers
Mechanical	Blume et al[27]	2008	RCT	342	NPWT vs moist wound therapy in diabetic foot ulcers
	Burke et al[28]	1998	RCT	42	Conservative treatment with whirlpool vs conservative treatment alone in stage III/IV pressure ulcers
	Eginton et al[21]	2003	RCT	7	NPWT vs moist wound therapy in diabetic foot wounds
	McCallon et al[22]	2000	RCT	10	VAC vs saline gauze in diabetic foot wounds
	Moues et al[24]	2004, 2006	RCT	54	VAC vs conventional gauze in chronic wounds
	Perez et al[25]	2010	RCT	40	Homemade VAC system vs saline dressings in complex wounds
	Wanner et al[26]	2003	RCT	22	VAC vs saline gauze in pressure sores
Enzymatic	Konig et al[31]	2005	RCT	42	Collagenase vs autolytic dressing in chronic leg ulcers
	Martin et al[32]	1996	RCT; double-blind	17	Streptokinase/streptodornase with hydrogel vs hydrogel alone in stage IV pressure ulcers
	Westerhof et al[29]	1987	RCT; double-blind	37	Fibrinolysin-desoxyribonuclease vs nonenzymatic treatment in chronic leg ulcers
	Westerhof et al[30]	1990	RCT; single-blind	31	Krill enzymes vs nonenzymatic treatment in venous leg ulcers
Autolytic	Brown-Etris et al[33]	2008	RCT	82	Transparent absorbent acrylic dressing vs hydrocolloid dressing in stage II/III pressure ulcers
	Gethin and Cowman[34]	2008	RCT; single-blind	108	Manuka honey vs hydrogel dressing in venous leg ulcers
	Kerihuel[35]	2010	RCT	119	Activated charcoal dressings vs hydrocolloid dressing in the chronic wounds
	Motta et al[36]	1999	RCT	10	Polymer hydrogel vs hydrocolloid in stage II/III pressure ulcers

Abbreviations: NPWT, negative pressure wound therapy; RCT, randomized controlled trial; VAC, vacuum-assisted closure.

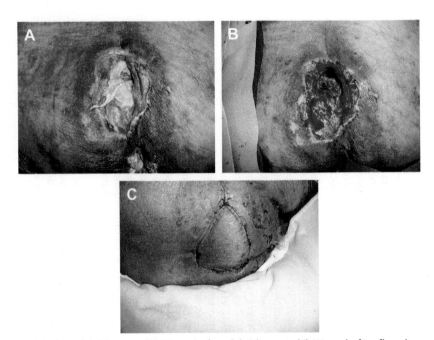

Fig. 1. (*A*) Wound before debridement. (*B*) Wound after debridement. (*C*) Wound after flap closure.

a multicenter trial. This finding could be explained by differences in experience dealing with chronic wounds among the trial centers.

A new technology has revolutionized surgical debridement: the high-powered parallel water jet tool (Versajet, Smith & Nephew Inc., Largo, FL, USA). This method has also been referred to as *tangential hydrosurgery*. A prospective randomized controlled trial was published in 2008 that compared this new tool with conventional surgical debridement in lower-extremity ulcers.[15] No significant difference in time to wound closure was found between the groups. Debridement time was significantly shorter in the hydrosurgery group by an average of 6.9 minutes. Ultimately, the benefits of hydrosurgery are difficult to quantify. This system allows far more precision, leading to the preparation of an adequate wound bed with less collateral tissue damage.

In summary, surgical debridement, whether sharp or through tangential hydrosurgery, provides the quickest and most complete method of debriding a wound. However, in patients with large wounds or other comorbidities, extensive surgery may not be feasible. The high-powered parallel water jet allows more precision in these patients but still necessitates a visit to the operating room, which requires adequate pain control, a sterile environment, and ensuring an adequate blood supply to the area being debrided.

Biologic Debridement

Biologic debridement is accomplished through the use of sterilized maggots, specifically from the larvae of the greenbottle fly (*Lucilia sericata*). A cohort-controlled study published in 2002 examined the difference between pressure ulcers treated with conventional therapy and those treated with maggot therapy.[16] Results showed that patients treated with maggot therapy experienced

- A greater number of completely debrided wounds
- A greater decrease in necrotic tissue
- A greater increase in granulation tissue
- A decrease in wound size.

Another more recent study discusses the management of wounds using freely mobile maggots or maggots contained in specialized bags that facilitate wound examination.[17]

One study was included that met the inclusion and exclusion criteria. The study was a derivative of the larval therapy Venous Ulcer Study[18] (VenUS II), which compared the efficacy of larval therapy and hydrogel debridement for sloughy or necrotic leg ulcers.[19] Results showed no difference in time to healing between the groups, but larval therapy significantly decreased the time to debridement. Health-related quality of life was not different between the groups.

A related study using the same set of patients compared the cost-effectiveness of larval therapy versus hydrogel debridement.[20] This study found no significant difference in the cost of larval therapy compared with hydrogel debridement; in fact, larval therapy on average was more costly than hydrogel debridement.

Biologic debridement has not gained wide-spread acceptance in the United States, likely because of patient and surgeon aversion. In Europe, however, biologic debridement is widely practiced.[17] Maggots are efficient and selective at digesting necrotic tissue and pathogens, and work fairly rapidly.

Mechanical Debridement

Mechanical debridement involves physical removal of necrotic tissue from a wound by means of:

- Wet-to-dry dressing changes
- Wound irrigation
- Hydrotherapy
- Negative pressure wound therapy (NPWT).

In general, these methods do not require patients to go to the operating room.

Comparison of wet-to-dry dressing changes and NPWT

The literature search revealed seven studies comparing the efficacy of wet-to-dry gauze dressings versus NPWT.[21–26] The first, published in 2000, examined the time to satisfactory healing and the change in wound surface area among the two modalities in the healing of surgically debrided diabetic foot wounds.[22] Results showed that satisfactory healing, calculated from the date of initial debridement to the date of definitive closure, was achieved in approximately half the time in the NPWT group, and a decrease in wound surface area was seen in the NPWT group compared with an increase in wound surface area in the saline-moistened gauze group. No mention was made of statistically significant findings in this study.

In 2003 a randomized controlled crossover study was published examining the wound dimensions and wound volume of surgically debrided diabetic foot wounds between NPWT and conventional dressings.[21] Results showed that NPWT significantly decreased the wound volume and depth compared with saline-moistened gauze.

That same year, another study examined the time it took to observe a 50% reduction in wound size between NPWT and conventional dressings in patients with surgically debrided pressure sores of the pelvic region.[26] No difference was found between the NPWT group and the conventional moist-gauze group. It was also noted that each method was effective in forming granulation tissue.

The next study, published in 2004, examined the effect of NPWT on bacterial load and wound surface area on surgically debrided wounds.[24] Results showed that NPWT significantly reduced

wound surface area by more than conventional moist-gauze therapy. In addition, a significant decrease in nonfermentative gram-negative bacilli and a significant increase in Staphylococcus aureus in the NPWT group were seen. The authors concluded that NPWT had a positive effect on wound healing, but that this effect was not explained by a reduction in bacterial load. A follow-up study using what seems to be the same patient set was published by the same authors in 2007.[23] The only additional information provided by this study was a tendency toward shorter duration of therapy in the NPWT group; ttwo wounds included in this patient set were traumatic in nature.

Variation on NPWT

A study comparing NPWT and traditional dressings presented an interesting variation on NPWT, using a homemade vacuum dressing system made from scrub brushes.[25] This study found that the homemade NPWT system significantly reduced healing time compared with traditional saline-soaked dressings. The homemade NPWT group received radical surgical debridement before therapy, whereas the control group received debridement if clinically indicated.

Comparison of NPWT and advanced moist wound therapy

Another study compared NPWT with advanced moist wound therapy (AMWT), defined as predominantly hydrogels and alginates, in the treatment of diabetic foot ulcers.[27] Results showed that ere a greater proportion of wounds achieved closure among the NPWT group. Furthermore, the NPWT group experienced fewer secondary amputations than the AMWT group.

Hydrotherapy

The final method of mechanical debridement examined was hydrotherapy, defined as whirlpool use, which was compared with traditional dressing changes in the treatment of pressure ulcers.[28] It was found that the group undergoing whirlpool therapy in addition to conservative treatment had a faster rate of improvement in wound dimensions.

Key conclusions on mechanical debridement

- Mechanical debridement is effective in removing surface eschar and debris.
- Mechanical debridement can often be painful to the patient when changing dressings.
- Granulation tissue that forms in the wound bed may be at risk during dressing changes.
- Although mechanical debridement is a relatively slow process, it can be effective

in chronic wounds in patients in whom other methods of debridement are contraindicated.

Enzymatic Debridement

Four studies examining enzymatic debridement were identified that met the inclusion/exclusion criteria.[29,30]

Comparison of fibrinolysin-desoxyribonuclease solution with saline solution

The first study compared the use of a fibrinolysin-desoxyribonuclease solution versus a saline solution for the debridement of chronic leg ulcers.[29] The enzymatic preparation was significantly more effective in debriding the wound, measured as percent of ulcer covered with debris, and formation of granulation tissue, measured as percent of wound covered with granulation tissue.

Comparison of krill enzyme with saline

The next study, by the same author, examined the efficacy of an enzyme present in the digestive system of the Antarctic krill (Euphausia superba) in the debridement of venous leg ulcers.[30] The enzymatic preparation was found to be significantly more effective than saline in cleansing the wound, measured using computer imaging of the wound examining areas of black and yellow necrosis.

Comparison of enzyme with autolytic dressing

Another study examined the use of collagenase compared with an autolytic dressing in the treatment of chronic leg ulcers.[31] The autolytic dressing seemed to be superior to the enzymatic preparation in the appearance of eschar/slough, granulation tissue, and reepithelialized area, but no significant difference was reported.

Efficacy of streptokinase/streptodornase in hydrogel

The final study compared the use of streptokinase/streptodornase in a hydrogel with the hydrogel alone in the management of stage IV pressure ulcers.[32] Results showed that fewer days were needed for eschar removal in the hydrogel-only group compared with the enzyme/hydrogel group, but this was not significant.

Key conclusions on enzymatic debridement

- Enzymatic debridement is useful for removal of moist and flimsy eschar and tissue debris but lacks the ability to penetrate thick eschar.
- The application may be painful to the patient.

Autolytic Debridement

Four studies examining autolytic debridement were identified that met the inclusion/exclusion criteria.[33–36]

The first study compared the efficacy of a polymer hydrogel and a hydrocolloid in the management of a pressure ulcer.[36] No significant difference in healing rate was noted between groups.

A study published in 2008 compared the efficacy of a transparent absorbent acrylic dressing with a hydrocolloid dressing in the treatment of pressure ulcers.[33] No difference was noted in wound closure rate and linear healing rate between the groups.

The next study compared the bacteriologic changes in venous leg ulcers treated with honey or a hydrogel.[34] Methicillin-resistant Staphylococcus aureus–positive wounds treated with manuka honey were found to be more likely to clear the infection than those treated with hydrogel.

The final study evaluating autolytic debridement assessed the effect of charcoal dressings compared with a hydrocolloid dressing on healing outcomes in chronic wounds.[35] No significant reduction in wound area was noted in either pressure ulcers or venous leg ulcers.

Dressings for leg and foot ulcers

A Cochrane Library systematic review was found on various dressings in the treatment of venous leg ulcers.[37] No significant differences were seen among dressings, and the authors recommend choosing dressing based on cost and physician preference. Another Cochrane Library systematic review regarding debridement of diabetic foot ulcers concluded that hydrogel use may result in faster healing than simple gauze dressings.[38]

Key conclusions on autolytic debridement

- Autolytic debridement promotes hydration of wounds and removal of tissue by the body's own enzymes.
- Wounds must be cleared of any remaining debris at each dressing change.

General Recommendations on Debridement

Evidence based medicine is a noble endeavor, but has its limits of efficacy with regard to wound debridement. Historical experience and the experience of most surgeons, wound care experts, and dermatologists show that wound healing can be achieved more readily with decreased morbidity when barriers to wound healing are removed, including bacteria, foreign bodies, tissue necrosis, moisture imbalances, and any condition that leads to an unfavorable wound milieu. Debridement in all forms facilitates the removal of these barriers and leads to improvement in wounds. Of the methods discussed, surgical debridement provides the fastest route to an appropriate wound bed and, barring any comorbidities, should be considered the standard of care in wound debridement. Other methods have more specific indications and should be used accordingly.

REFERENCES

1. Majno G. The healing hand: man and wound in the ancient world. Cambridge (MA): Harvard University Press; 1975.
2. Meade RH. An introduction to the history of general surgery. Philadelphia: Saunders; 1968.
3. Dobson J, Walker RM. Barbers and barber-surgeons of London: a history of the barbers' and barber-surgeons companies. Oxford (UK): Blackwell Scientific Publications for the Worshipful Company of Barbers; 1979.
4. Whipple AO. The story of wound healing and wound repair. Springfield (IL): Thomas; 1963.
5. Krizek T, Robson MC, Kho E. Bacterial growth and skin graft survival. Surg Forum 1967;18:518–9.
6. Granick MS, Tenenhaus M, Knox KR, et al. Comparison of wound irrigation and tangential hydrodissection in bacterial clearance of contaminated wounds: results of a randomized, controlled clinical study. Ostomy Wound Manage 2007;53(4):64–6, 68–70, 72.
7. Armstrong DG, Lavery LA. Clinical care of the diabetic foot. 2nd edition. Alexandria (VA): American Diabetes Association; 2010.
8. Baranoski S, Ayello EA. Wound care essentials: practice principles. 2nd edition. Philadelphia: Lippincott Williams & Wilkins; 2008.
9. Harper MS. Debridement. 1st edition. Garden City (NY): Doubleday; 1973.
10. Krasner D, Rodeheaver GT, Sibbald RG. Chronic wound care: a clinical source book for healthcare professionals. 4th edition. Malvern (PA): HMP Communications; 2007.
11. Granick MS, Gamelli RL. Surgical wound healing and management. New York: Informa Healthcare; 2007.
12. Schultz GS, Sibbald RG, Falanga V, et al. Wound bed preparation: a systematic approach to wound management. Wound Repair Regen 2003; 11(Suppl 1):S1–28.
13. Cardinal M, Eisenbud DE, Armstrong DG, et al. Serial surgical debridement: a retrospective study on clinical outcomes in chronic lower extremity wounds. Wound Repair Regen 2009;17(3):306–11.
14. Steed DL, Donohoe D, Webster MW, et al. Effect of extensive debridement and treatment on the healing of diabetic foot ulcers. Diabetic Ulcer Study Group. J Am Coll Surg 1996;183(1):61–4.
15. Caputo WJ, Beggs DJ, DeFede JL, et al. A prospective randomised controlled clinical trial comparing hydrosurgery debridement with conventional surgical debridement in lower extremity ulcers. Int Wound J 2008;5(2):288–94.
16. Sherman RA. Maggot versus conservative debridement therapy for the treatment of pressure ulcers. Wound Repair Regen 2002;10(4):208–14.
17. Gottrup F, Jorgensen B. Maggot debridement: an alternative method for debridement. Eplasty 2011; 11:e33.
18. Dumville JC, Worthy G, Soares MO, et al. VenUS II: a randomised controlled trial of larval therapy in the management of leg ulcers. Health Technol Assess 2009;13(55):1–182, iii–iv.
19. Dumville JC, Worthy G, Bland JM, et al. Larval therapy for leg ulcers (VenUS II): randomised controlled trial. BMJ 2009;338:b773.
20. Soares MO, Iglesias CP, Bland JM, et al. Cost effectiveness analysis of larval therapy for leg ulcers. BMJ 2009;338:b825.
21. Eginton MT, Brown KR, Seabrook GR, et al. A prospective randomized evaluation of negative-pressure wound dressings for diabetic foot wounds. Ann Vasc Surg 2003;17(6):645–9.
22. McCallon SK, Knight CA, Valiulus JP, et al. Vacuum-assisted closure versus saline-moistened gauze in the healing of postoperative diabetic foot wounds. Ostomy Wound Manage 2000;46(8):28–32, 34.
23. Moues CM, van den Bemd GJ, Heule F, et al. Comparing conventional gauze therapy to vacuum-assisted closure wound therapy: a prospective randomised trial. J Plast Reconstr Aesthet Surg 2007;60(6):672–81.
24. Moues CM, Vos MC, van den Bemd GJ, et al. Bacterial load in relation to vacuum-assisted closure wound therapy: a prospective randomized trial. Wound Repair Regen 2004;12(1):11–7.
25. Perez D, Bramkamp M, Exe C, et al. Modern wound care for the poor: a randomized clinical trial comparing the vacuum system with conventional saline-soaked gauze dressings. Am J Surg 2010; 199(1):14–20.
26. Wanner MB, Schwarzl F, Strub B, et al. Vacuum-assisted wound closure for cheaper and more comfortable healing of pressure sores: a prospective study. Scand J Plast Reconstr Surg Hand Surg 2003;37(1): 28–33.
27. Blume PA, Walters J, Payne W, et al. Comparison of negative pressure wound therapy using vacuum-assisted closure with advanced moist wound therapy in the treatment of diabetic foot ulcers: a multicenter randomized controlled trial. Diabetes Care 2008;31(4):631–6.
28. Burke DT, Ho CH, Saucier MA, et al. Effects of hydrotherapy on pressure ulcer healing. Am J Phys Med Rehabil 1998;77(5):394–8.

29. Westerhof W, Jansen FC, de Wit FS, et al. Controlled double-blind trial of fibrinolysin-desoxyribonuclease (Elase) solution in patients with chronic leg ulcers who are treated before autologous skin grafting. J Am Acad Dermatol 1987;17(1):32–9.

30. Westerhof W, van Ginkel CJ, Cohen EB, et al. Prospective randomized study comparing the debriding effect of krill enzymes and a non-enzymatic treatment in venous leg ulcers. Dermatologica 1990;181(4):293–7.

31. Konig M, Vanscheidt W, Augustin M, et al. Enzymatic versus autolytic debridement of chronic leg ulcers: a prospective randomised trial. J Wound Care 2005;14(7):320–3.

32. Martin SJ, Corrado OJ, Kay EA. Enzymatic debridement for necrotic wounds. J Wound Care 1996;5(7):310–1.

33. Brown-Etris M, Milne C, Orsted H, et al. A prospective, randomized, multisite clinical evaluation of a transparent absorbent acrylic dressing and a hydrocolloid dressing in the management of stage II and shallow Stage III pressure ulcers. Adv Skin Wound Care 2008;21(4):169–74.

34. Gethin G, Cowman S. Bacteriological changes in sloughy venous leg ulcers treated with manuka honey or hydrogel: an RCT. J Wound Care 2008; 17(6):241–4, 246–7.

35. Kerihuel JC. Effect of activated charcoal dressings on healing outcomes of chronic wounds. J Wound Care 2010;19(5):208, 210–2, 214–5.

36. Motta G, Dunham L, Dye T, et al. Clinical efficacy and cost-effectiveness of a new synthetic polymer sheet wound dressing. Ostomy Wound Manage 1999;45(10):41, 44–6, 48–9.

37. Palfreyman SJ, Nelson EA, Lochiel R, et al. Dressings for healing venous leg ulcers. Cochrane Database Syst Rev 2006;(3):CD001103.

38. Edwards J, Stapley S. Debridement of diabetic foot ulcers. Cochrane Database Syst Rev 2010;1:CD003556.

Microbial Barriers

Luke G. Gutwein, MD[a], Mousumee Panigrahi, BS[a],
Gregory S. Schultz, PhD[b], Bruce A. Mast, MD[a],*

KEYWORDS

- Barrier therapy • Wound healing • Biofilms • Acute wounds • Chronic wounds

KEY POINTS

- The wound healing process can be hindered easily by the bacterial bioburden with organized and dynamic polymicrobial biofilms.
- For new or acute wounds, the use of an appropriate dressing that acts as a microbial barrier is essential.
- For delayed-healing or chronic wounds, adequate sharp debridement when clinically indicated is imperative as the initial step to break the imbalanced cellular microenvironment–bioburden cycle.
- Adjunctive microbial barriers act to minimize bacterial contamination from the environment and facilitate the conversion of the chronic wound to an acute wound, which ultimately leads to a healed wound.

INTRODUCTION

Wound care has evolved over thousands of year from an archaic therapy of honey, grease, and lint[1] to an inconceivable use of modern health care resources. Each wound infection may cost up to $35,000 to treat,[2] and the annual cost of pressure ulcers alone mounts to billions of dollars.[3] In 1865, Sir Joseph Lister was the first to understand and implement an antimicrobial wound therapy.[4] Antiseptic carbolic acid (phenol) demonstrated improved wound healing without suppuration and reduced mortality. During World War I, Alexis Carrel treated open wounds with sodium hypochlorite (Dakin solution), which aided necrotic debridement of devitalized tissue.[5] Today the wound market is replete with innovative technological advances for wound care including technology that helps prevent infection by antimicrobial barrier therapy. This article reviews the complexities of bacteria and wound healing, the current application of antimicrobial wound therapy, and pioneering advances in wound care technology.

WOUND HEALING
Acute Wounds

An acute wound is created by a violation in skin integrity. Acute wound healing progresses through a systematic and balanced repair process consisting of 4 phases: (1) hemostasis, (2) inflammation, (3) proliferation, and (4) remodeling.

The hemostatic phase is initiated immediately upon injury, characterized by both the intrinsic and extrinsic clotting cascades. When an injury occurs, collagen, Von Willibrand factor, and tissue factor are exposed from the subendothelium to the blood stream, acting as the inciting catalyst for the systematic repair process. A platelet plug forms, composed of platelets and fibrin. Platelets release granules containing multiple growth factors acting as a chemoattractant and thromboxane A2 acting as a potent vasoconstrictor. Transforming growth factor-beta (TGF-β) is the key growth factor released, playing a central role in wound healing.[6]

The inflammatory phase from days 1 to 10 is characterized by an inflammatory cell wound infiltration

[a] Division of Plastic & Reconstructive Surgery, Department of Surgery, University of Florida, Post Office Box 100286, 1600 Southwest Archer Road, Gainesville, FL 32610, USA; [b] Department of Obstetrics and Gynecology, Institute for Wound Research, Room M337F, 1600 Southwest Archer Road, University of Florida, Gainesville, FL 32610-0294, USA
* Corresponding author.
E-mail address: Bruce.Mast@surgery.ufl.edu

Clin Plastic Surg 39 (2012) 229–238
doi:10.1016/j.cps.2012.04.002
0094-1298/12/$ – see front matter © 2012 Elsevier Inc. All rights reserved.

and initiation of epithelialization occurring at 1 to 2 mm/d from wound edges. The ordered cellular influx begins with neutrophils that act as scavengers cleaning the cellular debris through phagocytosis and killing bacteria through the oxidative burst. Neutrophils secrete elastase and matrix metalloproteinases (MMPs) to degrade extracellular matrix (ECM), facilitating cellular migration.[6] Monocytes from the blood convert to macrophages arriving at 48 hours, which are the key coordinating cells for transitioning to the proliferative phase by releasing additional growth factors and mediating angiogenesis, fibroplasia, and synthesizing nitric oxide.[7]

From day 5, fibroblasts arrive at the wound, initiating the proliferative phase. Type 3 collagen deposition, neovascularization, and granulation tissue characterize the proliferative phase. Granulation tissue is perfused connective tissue allowing the framework for further epithelialization. Fibroblasts in the wound convert to myofibroblasts to allow wound contraction, which is the key component for healing via secondary intention. Cellular signaling for this conversion is mediated by macrophages through TGF-β.[8] Fibroblasts also secrete MMP, which aids to facilitating cellular migration.

From day 8 through year 1, wound remodeling and maturation occur. Initial deposition of collagen is disordered, and over time remodeling of collagen at areas of increased stress allow for increased tensile strength. By week 3, type 3 collagen has been exchanged for type 1 collagen, which is the most common type of collagen in the human body. The maximal tensile strength is reached at approximately 8 weeks after injury, at 80% of its original strength. Key local wound factors to sustain a systematic repair process are listed in **Box 1**.

Three main components required for normal wound healing[6] are (1) connective tissue deposition, (2) contraction, and (3) epithelialization.

Depending on the wound closure mechanism, one component may contribute further to the systematic repair process. For example, in primary closure, wound healing is chiefly dependent on connective tissue deposition. Mechanical forces provided by foreign bodies (suture, staples, adhesive) aid in contracture. In secondary intention, wound closure is highly dependent on contraction and connective tissue deposition. Lastly, a donor site of a split-thickness skin graft heals principally from epithelialization via the wound margin or residual skin appendages located within the remaining reticular dermis.

Chronic Wounds

When the ordered repair process fails, an acute wound is converted to a chronic wound. There is an imbalance in the cellular microenvironment, disrupting normal production and degradation steps (**Fig. 1**). Often, chronic wounds are a manifestation of other comorbidities, particularly in a poor nutritional state. There are multiple etiologies of a chronic wound, and a common theme among all chronic wounds is the bacterial bioburden (**Fig. 2**). A chronic wound is subjected to the inflammatory phase indefinitely, which inhibits granulation tissue formation, a prerequisite for contraction and epithelialization. Chronic wounds demonstrate a higher level of proinflammatory cytokines and fewer mitogenic cells.[9–13] Fibroblasts convert to a senescent state, delaying the proliferative phase.[14] In order for granulation tissue to form, nutrients and substrates must be available. Neovascularization is required; however, with an imbalance of ECM proteins, growth factors, MMPs, and protease inhibitors, the formation of an organized vascular network is delayed. A delay in healing allows bacterial contamination, which can further cause an imbalanced cellular microenvironment (**Fig. 3**).

Reducing the bacterial bioburden is a key step in healing a chronic wound. Sharp debridement removes nonviable tissue and frequently a significant degree of bioburden, but also provides conversion of a chronic wound to an acute wound.[3] Often multiple debridement sessions are required to optimize wound healing conditions. Essential adjuncts to sharp debridement are microbial barriers that function to prevent bacterial contamination and infection. Once applied, microbial barriers act to restore a proper balance to the cellular microenvironment.

BACTERIAL IMPACT ON WOUND HEALING

Bacteria colonize a wound within 48 hours.[15] Most bacteria have low virulence and do not invade the tissue. Invasive species include *Pseudomonas aeruginosa, Staphylococcus aureus, Streptococcus,* and *Clostridium.* The wound relation with

---

Box 1
Local factors that affect wound healing

1. Ensure a moist environment
2. Optimize O_2 delivery
3. Minimize edema through compression
4. Adequate debridement to remove necrotic tissue
5. Avoid infection
6. Limit foreign bodies
7. Microbial barrier therapy

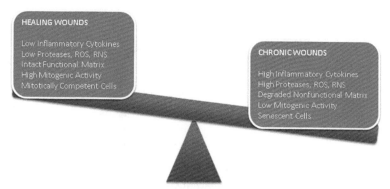

Fig. 1. There is an imbalanced cellular microenvironment between healing wounds and chronic wounds. Chronic wounds have an increased inflammatory state. ROS, reactive oxygen species; RNS, reactive nitrogen species.

bacteria consists of a continuum from contamination to wound septicemia. Contamination within a wound is defined by nonreplicating bacteria.[16,17] Colonization within a wound is defined as replicating bacteria adherent to the wound without tissue damage.[16,17] Colonization does not delay wound healing. However, critical colonization, which is a transition state from colonization to invasive wound infection, may delay wound healing.[16,17] The virulence and the amount of bacteria in the wound determine progression to tissue invasion. Once host tissue destruction occurs by replicating bacteria, a wound infection is present. Historically, 1.0×10^5 bacteria per gram of tissue is the necessary amount of bacteria to interrupt the wound healing process. This is determined by tissue biopsy and quantitative culture, which comprise the gold standard for diagnosis. However, it is commonplace to diagnose bacterial wound infections based on clinical signs of exudate and inflammation (warmth, edema, erythema, and pain), forgoing tissue biopsy and quantitative culture. Recently, the 1.0×10^5 bacteria per gram of tissue has been called into question.[16] Virulence among bacteria differs by species. Therefore, the bacteria load required for tissue destruction differs by species. Additionally, synergism among organisms will inhibit wound healing potently as compared with a single organism. The presence of 4 or more different bacterial species correlates with delayed wound healing.[18–20]

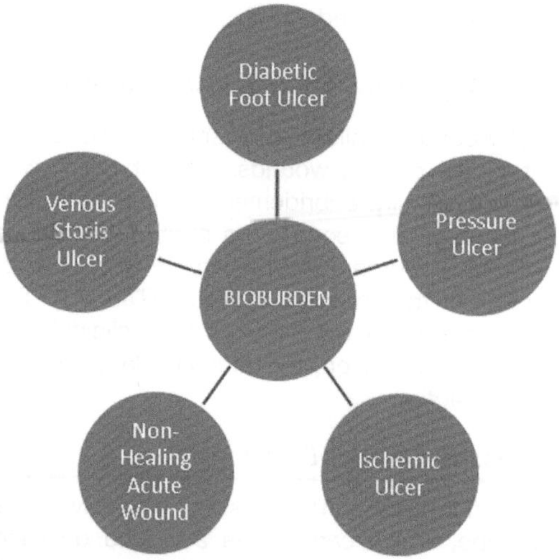

Bacterial organization differs among acute wound infection and chronic wound infection.[21]

- In acute wounds, bacteria exist as free-floating planktonic organisms and must be rapidly controlled to prevent tissue destruction and wound sepsis.
- Bacteria in chronic wounds do not exist as planktonic organisms but rather as biofilms able to resist the host inflammatory cascade and antibiotic therapy.[22,23]

BIOFILMS AS BARRIERS IN WOUND HEALING

Biofilms are a principal impediment to healing chronic wounds.[16,24,25] The extracellular polysaccharide matrix (EPS) provides an aggregation community for bacteria to evade the host immune response, resist systemic antibiotics, and facilitate plasmid transfer leading to highly virulent organisms.[16,23,26] Biofilms increase the antibiotic minimum inhibitory concentration 1000 times that of planktonic bacteria.[26] External to the plasma membrane, all cells have a glycocalyx, including bacteria. The bacterial glycocalyx interacts with

Fig. 2. The etiology of chronic wounds is multifactorial and dependent on the nutritional state and co-morbidities. A common motif of chronic wounds is the bacterial bioburden.

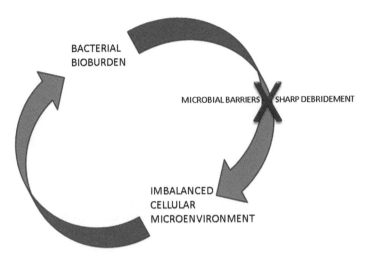

BACTERIAL BIOBURDEN

MICROBIAL BARRIERS   SHARP DEBRIDEMENT

IMBALANCED CELLULAR MICROENVIRONMENT

Fig. 3. The perpetual cycle between bioburden and an imbalanced cellular microenvironment is essential to break. Adequate debridement is imperative, and microbial barriers aid as an adjunct to minimize the bioburden.

the bacterial secreted EPS, allowing a sessile morphology of the community bacterial aggregate. Acting as a barrier, the EPS is effective at inhibiting host phagocytic cell penetration. Native biofilms are present on the skin, genitourinary tracts, intestine, and respiratory epithelium.[23] Biofilms have been encountered in various diseases such as osteomyelitis, cystic fibrosis, and endocarditis.[27] They also form on indwelling foreign material such as urinary catheters, endotracheal tubes, and prosthetic implants. In wounds, biofilms occur at a liquid tissue interface and induce a state of chronic inflammation, delaying the wound healing processs.[24] The moist environment of a chronic wound with abundant nutrients provides the ideal habitat for bacteria to form a biofilm.[24] James and colleagues[28] demonstrated that biofilms are prevalent among chronic wounds (60% of biopsied chronic wounds) but rare among acute wounds (6% of biopsied acute wounds).

In normal wound healing, neutrophils arrive, initiating the inflammatory phase of wound healing within hours of wound formation. Reactive oxygen species secreted by the neutrophils provide cellular defense against bacteria. Jesaitis and colleagues[29] demonstrated that this oxidative burst is attenuated 50% to 80% by the presence of biofilms. Biofilms also inhibit phagocytosis by interfering with efficient complement opsonization of bacteria.[23] Biofilms consist of a dynamic microbial population. James and colleagues[28] demonstrated that chronic wound biofilms are polymicrobial, commonly including *Staphylococcus aureus*, *Enterococcus faecalis*, and *Pseudomonas aeruginosa*. The polymicrobial nature facilitates delayed wound healing because of the large array of genetic diversity among the multiple bacterial species. In

addition, biofilm growth exhibits an increased level of mutations.[27] Biofilms are difficult to treat effectively and arrest the wound in chronic inflammation. Surgical removal of the biofilm is presently the most effective treatment modality. Wolcott and colleagues[30] demonstrated that within 72 hours of wound debridement, bacterial susceptibility was significantly increased to antimicrobial therapy. However, after 72 hours, mature biofilms had reconstituted a resistant phenotype. Microbial barrier therapy is playing an increasingly important role in actively fighting against biofilms and bioburden inherent to chronic wounds. Barrier therapy is also used in acute wounds to aid in prevention of infection and biofilm formation. Many antimicrobial barrier wound therapies exist as an adjunct to apply after adequate debridement.

MICROBIAL BARRIER WOUND THERAPY

Most wounds applicable for antimicrobial barrier therapy are chronic wounds. In combination with aggressive sharp debridement, antimicrobial barrier therapy has become the strategy to reduce bacterial bioburden and biofilm.[3,30] Many microbial barrier methods are available (**Table 1**). The following section will highlight their clinical use, mechanism of action, and, if available, evidence-based practice.

The Passive Barrier Dressings

A commonplace barrier dressing is simply gauze and tape, which can act as a wound dressing for acute or chronic wounds. In an acute wound, gauze works especially well if there is little drainage. It is typically removed 48 hours after primary wound closure, the time needed for wound

Table 1
Microbial barrier therapy characteristics

Wound Barrier Type	Barrier Strength	Removal	Antimicrobial
Gauze	+	+	0
Bioguard	++	+	+++
Polyurethane film (Tegaderm, Opsite)	++	0	0
Tegaderm CHG	++	0	++
Dermabond®	+++	0	++
Telfa	+	0	0
Telfa PHMB	+	0	++
Alginate	+	+	0
Hydrocolloid	+	+	0
Hydrofiber	+	+	0
Foam	+	+	0
Ag VAC Sponge	+++	+++	++
Ag Foam	+	+	++
Ag Alginate	+	+	++
Ag Hydrocolloid	+	+	++
Acticoat	+	0	++
Aquacel Ag	+	0	++
Biopatch	+	0	++
Iodine gel pad	+	+	++

Abbreviations: Ag, silver; CHG, chlorhexadine gluconate; PHMB, polyhexamethylene biguanide.

epithelialization. In this manner, the gauze is simply a barrier to the external environment, minimizing possible contamination. In the interim, if the gauze becomes saturated, the skin margins are at risk for maceration. If this occurs within 48 hours of primary wound closure, the saturated gauze should be changed.

For chronic wounds, bulk gauze functions to absorb and control wound exudate. Again, once the gauze is saturated, the dressing should be changed. A moist rather than a desiccated wound is the ideal environment for wound healing; however, excessive fluid promotes bacterial viability and inhibits wound healing. Moistened gauze dressing changes are required at a minimum 2 to 3 times per day depending on local wound conditions. The advantage of moistened gauze dressing changes includes microdebridement, as the gauze is removed from the wound bed. There are disadvantages to dressing changes[15]:

1. Microdebridement caused by gauze removal is indiscriminatory and removes healthy granulation tissue as well
2. Tissue necrosis occurs if the gauze is packed too tightly
3. There is a prolonged inflammatory state
4. Dressing changes are labor-intensive
5. They are often painful for patients.

Additional barrier dressings with absorptive capacity include alginate, hydrofiber, and foam dressings. All 3 dressings function in a similar manner to absorb wound exudate and require less frequent dressing changes from simple gauze. Alginate derived from seaweed exchanges the sodium in the wound exudate for calcium, which aids in hemostasis after debridement. Hydrofiber dressings absorb exudate and transform into a gel at the wound surface. Polyurethane foam dressings allow a non-debridement removal from the wound and skin interface.

Hydrofiber dressings absorb exudate and transform into a gel at the wound surface.

Polyurethane film dressings (Tegaderm; 3 M, St. Paul, MN, USA) (Opsite; Smith & Nephew, Hull, UK) are gas-permeable and act to keep the right balance of moisture at the wound while protecting from external debris and fluids. Film dressings function well for wounds with little exudate while allowing evaporation of moisture accumulating under the dressing. They are well tolerated by patients secondary to the pliable nature and allow visible assessment of the wound or catheter site. Film dressings are commonly used at intravenous catheter sites and in combination with gauze at surgical sites. In addition, film dressings used at split-thickness skin graft donor sites have been associated with decreased pain.[31]

2-Octyl Cyanoacrylate Wound Films

Traditional use of the passive barrier dressing to prevent contamination and infection has evolved. The ideal dressing postoperative or post-dermal repair is impervious to bacterial contamination from the environment. First introduced in 1959, cyanoacrylates (methyl- and ethyl-2-cyanoacrylates) were implemented for skin closure, fixation of implants, closure of cerebrospinal fluid leaks, and tissue adhesion.[32–35] Cyanoacrylates did not gain popularity due to histotoxicity from the byproducts cyanoacetate and formaldehyde.[36,37] However, longer-chained molecules based from the cyanoacrylate formulation (Dermabond®; Ethicon, Somerville, NJ, USA and Indermil®; Covidien, Mansfield, MA, USA) have a slower degradation rate which decreases the concentration of byproducts in the tissue causing less inflammation allowing tissue biocompatibility.[33,34]

2-octyl cyanoacrylate formulations are excellent tissue adhesives due to their inherent characteristics when applied to tissue (**Box 2**). The barrier property of 2-octyl cyanoacrylate has been studied extensively clinically[33,38–41] and experimentally.[9,34,42,43] It has long been recognized that the more adherent an occlusive wound dressing, the better the dressing acts as a barrier to external contamination.[43,44] Narang and colleagues[34] demonstrated that an inoculum of numerous different test organisms could not penetrate a 2-octyl cyanoacrylate film. Over a 7-day period, the film depressed in agar medium was impervious to organisms. Positive control substituted sterile filter paper and demonstrated growth of every organism tested. Furthermore, 2-octyl cyanoacrylate has also been investigated for its antimicrobial properties. Mertz and colleagues demonstrated at 72 hours from animal wounding the superior antimicrobial ability of 2-octyl cyanoacrylate relative to 3 other treatment groups: standard bandage, hydrocolloid bandage, and no bandage (air-exposed). After wounding and inoculation of the wounds with *Pseudomonas aeruginosa* or *Staphylococcus aureus*, treatment groups were randomly assigned. Bacterial quantification after treatment bandages were removed in 72 hours discovered the 2-octyl cyanoacrylate to be significantly lower than the remaining 3 treatment groups, with the hydrocolloid dressing harboring the highest bacterial colonies. It is compelling that 2-octyl cyanoacrylate may have antimicrobial properties; however, no mechanism has been elucidated.

Formulations of 2-octyl cyanoacrylate are ubiquitous in operating rooms and have increased efficiency for wound closure while enhancing quality wound care and eliminating suture or staple removal.[33] Interestingly, clinical studies have not proven a congruent difference in cosmesis or wound infection rate as compared with adhesive strips[40] or skin staples.[39]

Silver-Impregnated Wound Therapy

Moyer and colleagues[45] were the first to report the antimicrobial effect of silver in 1965. An explosion of the silver-impregnated dressing market has occurred with an array of options. Although several forms are available—mesh, hydrocolloid, hydrogel, powder, foam, and polymeric film—fundamentally, all the formulations function in the same manner. In metallic form, silver is inert with no antimicrobial action. In solution, silver ionizes and becomes an extremely reactive cation. Silver has multiple sites of action on bacteria, including the cell wall, protein alteration, and binding to DNA to inhibit transcription.[3] Silver-impregnated dressings differ in their composition and application length of time. Acticoat (Smith & Nephew, Hull, UK) meshes nanocrystalline silver into rayon and polyester. The nanocrystalline structure provides expansive surface area for moisture contact, allowing silver to solubilize. Silver metal will not dissolve in solution however nanocrystalline silver is soluble with a concentration of 70 ppm.[3] This allows a sustained release of silver up to 7 days.[46] Aquacel Ag (Convatec, Skillman, NJ, USA) is composed of sodium carboxymethylcellulose, which forms a gel when exposed to wound moisture,

---

Box 2
Properties of Dermabond® (2-octyl cyanoacrylate)

1. Long shelf life
2. Polymerizes rapidly upon skin contact
3. Bonds to skin (2.5 minutes to maximum bond strength)
4. Strength equivalent to healed tissue at 7 days after repair
5. Biocompatible
6. Forms a flexible/nonbrittle film
7. Easily removed after healing/sloughs off upon turnover of skin
8. Does not impede wound healing
9. Increases epithelialization rate

promoting the wound healing microenvironment and retaining exudate. Acticoat and Aquacel Ag fundamentally differ in their quantity and release of silver. The silver content of Acticoat and Aquacel Ag is 109 and 19.7 mg/cm^2, respectively.[47] Aquacel Ag incorporates ionic silver in a hydrofiber mesh, whereas Acticoat incorporates nanocrystalline silver designed to ionize.[3,47]

The efficacy of silver-impregnated dressings has been established in vitro with bacteria in planktonic or biofilm model states.[48–50] Furthermore, Percival and colleagues[49] have advanced the in vitro testing field by establishing a flow cytometry wound model able to quantify between dead and live bacteria. Despite this, there is no substitute for clinical evidence-based medicine. Very few reports of randomized controlled trials exist evaluating the efficacy of silver-impregnated dressings compared with conventional wound dressings.[3,51] Khundkar and colleagues identified 31 studies applying Acticoat to burn wounds. Out of the 31 studies, only one randomized controlled trial exists that met qualifications for level 1 evidence that compared Acticoat against silver sulfadiazine. Sixty-five percent of studies were level 5 evidence. Aquacel Ag has been studied in application for burn patients. Literature does indicate a consensus that Aquacel Ag demonstrates financial and therapeutic benefit to burn patients.[52,53] Aquacel Ag may be changed every 2 to 3 days, whereas silver sulfadiazine requires daily dressing changes.

There is potential toxicity from silver-impregnated dressings; however, systemic absorption is rare if use is limited to less than 4 weeks and a wound area less than 30% total body surface area is covered. Local cytotoxicity of keratinocytes was studied by Paddle-Ledinek and colleagues.[47] Nine different wound dressing extracts were tested with keratinocyte cultures. Extracts of 4 different silver-impregnated dressings demonstrated the most disordered morphology and greatest cytotoxicity. The authors concluded that silver-impregnated dressings should be used with caution and are not advisable unless wound infection is a significant risk.

Negative-Pressure Wound Therapy

Since 1995, negative-pressure wound therapy (VAC; KCI, San Antonio, Texas) or vacuum-assisted closure (VAC) has grown increasingly popular for a microbial barrier and wound healing. VAC therapy has 2 primary identified mechanisms of action that aid in wound healing. Removing excess wound fluid or interstitial edema results from the increased pressure gradient created by the VAC. Local tissue pressure decreases, allowing capillaries to reperfuse.[54] Angiogenesis is up-regulated with increased capillary density and diameter in experimental models.[55] The second mechanism is mechanical deformation of cells created by the negative-pressure therapy. Soft tissue is viscoelastic and will deform slowly to mechanical forces over time.[54,56] Mechanical deformation causes cellular shear stress, which has been implicated in up-regulating vascular endothelial growth factor.[57] The amount of tissue deformation is critical and has been evaluated by Morykwas and colleagues. Their investigation entailed evaluating an animal wound closure model at different negative-pressure settings of 25, 125, and 500 mmHg. After 8 days of negative pressure, swine wounds were 21%, completely flush (ideal outcome), and 5.9% changed in defect volume at 25, 125, and 500 mmHg, respectively. Their postulated mechanism was that tissue deformation was too high at 500 mmHg resulting in poor perfusion with consequent 5.9% change in defect volume. Additionally, tissue deformation was minimal at the low negative pressure of at 25 mmHg with a change in defect volume of 21%.

Bacterial bioburden in animal studies has been found to decrease with VAC therapy.[58] However, clinical studies find that there is no decrease in bacterial bioburden with VAC therapy.[59,60] Moues and colleagues found in a randomized controlled trial comparing VAC therapy with moistened gauze therapy that there was a significant decrease in wound surface area but that wound biopsies demonstrated no significant difference in the bacterial load.[59] Furthermore, Weed and colleagues[60] performed a retrospective review from wounds that had a history quantitative culture swabs before, during, and after VAC therapy. Interestingly, the bacterial load was significantly higher during VAC therapy than before or after VAC therapy. Despite the recognized design flaws[54] in the retrospective study, 2 explanations may exist to explain why bacterial load may increase with VAC therapy in these studies. VAC sponges are recommended by the manufacturer to be changed every 3 to 5 days in clinical use. Changing the VAC more frequently will reduce bacterial load but may be of no clinical benefit. Additionally it is labor intensive, and cost ineffective. Furthermore, debridement of necrotic tissue is imperative before placement of VAC therapy. Without adequate debridement of devitalized tissue, the bacterial load will be increased.

Numerous other qualities as consequence of the local negative pressure created by the VAC have been discovered clinically or experimentally. VAC therapy has been recognized to salvage free tissue flaps from venous congestion,[61] decrease the serum myoglobin concentration in crush injuries,[62] increase the re-epithelialization rate of split thickness skin graft donor sites,[63] and decrease the zone of stasis progression to full thickness associated with thermal burn injury.[54,64]

The literature is replete with studies demonstrating the overall wound healing efficacy of the VAC in controlled experimental environments; however, there is an incongruent pattern clinically. This is best identified by a systematic review of randomized controlled trials[65] highlighting heterogeneity between trials and within trials responsible for the lack of agreement. Variation among trial endpoints and size and location of wounds makes direct comparison difficult to prove overall efficacy of the VAC in clinical trials. The authors concluded that with the current state of available evidence, VAC therapy is neither superior nor inferior as compared with conventional saline-moistened gauze.

BIOGUARD

Conventional antimicrobial barriers function to leach an impregnated histotoxic chemical (ie, silver ions, chlorhexidine, iodine, or polyhexamethylene biguanide) that is temporarily bound to the dressing. Recently approved by the US Food and Drug Administration, Bioguard (Derma Sciences, Princeton, NJ, USA) incorporates a permanently bound high molecular weight polycationic polymer. The polymer consists of concentrated positively charged quarternary amines that function to disrupt the bacterial membrane without leaching into the wound bed, disturbing the cellular microenvronment. In vitro cellular analysis has demonstrated a smaller zone of inhibition and improved cellular morphology at the Bioguard interface as compared with a silver-impregnated dressing.[66] Furthermore, Bioguard may eliminate potential bacterial resistance due to the inability of the functional group to be internalized by bacteria. Clinical observations from a burn unit with highly exudative wounds demonstrated that Bioguard gauze dressings were associated with no odor or metallic green staining (*Pseudomonas aeruginosa*) when compared with conventional gauze dressings, which did demonstrate odor and metallic green staining.[67]

SUMMARY

Wound healing is a complex systematic process that depends on multiple local and systemic factors. The wound healing process can easily be hindered by the bacterial bioburden with organized and dynamic polymicrobial biofilms. For new or acute wounds, the use of an appropriate dressing that acts as a microbial barrier is essential. For delayed-healing or chronic wounds, adequate sharp debridement when clinically indicated is imperative as the initial step to break the imbalanced cellular microenvironment–bioburden cycle. Adjunctive microbial barriers act to minimize bacterial contamination from the environment and facilitate the conversion of a chronic wound to an acute wound, which ultimately leads to a healed wound. There are a multitude of microbial barriers clinically available. Proper selection depends on wound behavior and location. Properly designed randomized clinical trials continue to play an integrated role in clinical care to prove efficacy of pioneering wound therapy.

REFERENCES

1. Broughton G 2nd, Janis JE, Attinger CE. A brief history of wound care. Plast Reconstr Surg 2006; 117:6S–11S.
2. Scott R. The direct medical costs of health care associated infections in US hospitals and the benefits of prevention. Atlanta (GA): Division of Healthcare Quality Promotion, National Center for Preparedness, Detection, and Control of Infectious Diseases, Coordinating Center for Infectious Diseases, Centers for Disease Control and Prevention; 2009.
3. Toy LW, Macera L. Evidence-based review of silver dressing use on chronic wounds. J Am Acad Nurse Pract 2011;23:183–92.
4. Lister BJ. The classic: on the antiseptic principle in the practice of surgery. 1867. Clin Orthop Relat Res 2010;468:2012–6.
5. Carrell A, Dehelly G. The treatment of infected wounds. New York: Hoeber; 1917.
6. Goldberg SR, Diegelmann RF. Wound healing primer. Surg Clin North Am 2010;90:1133–46.
7. Witte MB, Barbul A. Role of nitric oxide in wound repair. Am J Surg 2002;183:406–12.
8. Broughton G 2nd, Janis JE, Attinger CE. Wound healing: an overview. Plast Reconstr Surg 2006; 117:1e-S–32e-S.
9. Bhende S, Rothenburger S, Spangler DJ, et al. In vitro assessment of microbial barrier properties of Dermabond topical skin adhesive. Surg Infect (Larchmt) 2002;3:251–7.
10. Mast BA, Schultz GS. Interactions of cytokines, growth factors, and proteases in acute and chronic wounds. Wound Repair Regen 1996;4:411–20.
11. Yager DR, Chen SM, Ward S. The ability of chronic wound fluids to degrade peptide growth factors is associated with increased levels of elastase activity

and diminished levels of proteinase inhibitors. Wound Repair Regen 1997;81:23–32.

12. Yager DR, Nwomeh BC. The proteolytic environment of chronic wounds. Wound Repair Regen 1999;7: 433–41.

13. Yager DR, Zhang LY, Liang HX. Wound fluids from human pressure ulcers contain elevated matrix metalloproteinase levels and activity compared to surgical wound fluids. J Invest Dermatol 1996;107:743–8.

14. Harding KG, Moore K, Phillips TJ. Wound chronicity and fibroblast senescence—implications for treatment. Int Wound J 2005;2:364–8.

15. Krasner DL, Rodeheaver GT, Sibbald RG. Chronic wound care: a clinical source book for healthcare professionals. Malvern (PA): HMP Communications; 2007.

16. Edwards R, Harding KG. Bacteria and wound healing. Curr Opin Infect Dis 2004;17:91–6.

17. Landis SJ. Chronic wound infection and antimicrobial use. Adv Skin Wound Care 2008;21:531–40 [quiz: 541–2].

18. Bowler PG. The 10(5) bacterial growth guideline: reassessing its clinical relevance in wound healing. Ostomy Wound Manage 2003;49:44–53.

19. Hill KE, Davies CE, Newcombe RG, et al. A prospective characterization of the microbiology of chronic venous leg ulcers: the clinical predictive value of tissue biopsies and swabs re-evaluated [abstract]. Wound Repair Regen 2003;11(5):A1–54.

20. Trengove NJ, Stacey MC, McGechie DF, et al. Qualitative bacteriology and leg ulcer healing. J Wound Care 1996;5:277–80.

21. Wolcott R, Dowd S. The role of biofilms: are we hitting the right target? Plast Reconstr Surg 2011; 127(Suppl 1):28S–35S.

22. Phillips P, Sampson E, Yang O, et al. Bacterial biofilms in wounds. Wound Healing South Africa 2008;1:1–3.

23. Thomson CH. Biofilms: do they affect wound healing? Int Wound J 2011;8:63–7.

24. Percival SL, Hill KE, Malic S, et al. Antimicrobial tolerance and the significance of persister cells in recalcitrant chronic wound biofilms. Wound Repair Regen 2011;19:1–9.

25. Phillips PL, Yang Q, Sampson E, et al. Effects of antimicrobial agents on an in vitro biofilm model of skim wounds. Adv Wound Care 2010;1:299–304.

26. Chen L, Wen YM. The role of bacterial biofilm in persistent infections and control strategies. Int J Oral Sci 2011;3:66–73.

27. Hoiby N, Ciofu O, Johansen HK, et al. The clinical impact of bacterial biofilms. Int J Oral Sci 2011;3: 55–65.

28. James GA, Swogger E, Wolcott R, et al. Biofilms in chronic wounds. Wound Repair Regen 2008;16: 37–44.

29. Jesaitis AJ, Franklin MJ, Berglund D, et al. Compromised host defense on *Pseudomonas aeruginosa*

biofilms: characterization of neutrophil and biofilm interactions. J Immunol 2003;171:4329–39.

30. Wolcott RD, Rumbaugh KP, James G, et al. Biofilm maturity studies indicate sharp debridement opens a time-dependent therapeutic window. J Wound Care 2010;19:320–8.

31. Dornseifer U, Lonic D, Gerstung TI, et al. The ideal split-thickness skin graft donor-site dressing: a clinical comparative trial of a modified polyurethane dressing and Aquacel. Plast Reconstr Surg 2011; 128:918–24.

32. DeBono R. A simple, inexpensive method for precise application of cyanoacrylate tissue adhesive. Plast Reconstr Surg 1997;100:447–50.

33. Magee WP Jr, Ajkay N, Githae B, et al. Use of octyl-2-cyanoacrylate in cleft lip repair. Ann Plast Surg 2003;50:1–5.

34. Narang U, Mainwaring L, Spath G, et al. In-vitro analysis for microbial barrier properties of 2-octyl cyanoacrylate-derived wound treatment films. J Cutan Med Surg 2003;7:13–9.

35. Toriumi DM, O'Grady K, Desai D, et al. Use of octyl-2-cyanoacrylate for skin closure in facial plastic surgery. Plast Reconstr Surg 1998;102:2209–19.

36. Toriumi DM, Raslan WF, Friedman M, et al. Histotoxicity of cyanoacrylate tissue adhesives. A comparative study. Arch Otolaryngol Head Neck Surg 1990; 116:546–50.

37. Toriumi DM, Raslan WF, Friedman M, et al. Variable histotoxicity of histoacryl when used in a subcutaneous site: an experimental study. Laryngoscope 1991;101:339–43.

38. Carr JA. The intracorporeal use of 2-octyl cyanoacrylate resin to control air leaks after lung resection. Eur J Cardiothorac Surg 2011;39:579–83.

39. Ong J, Ho KS, Chew MH, et al. Prospective randomised study to evaluate the use of Dermabond ProPen (2-octylcyanoacrylate) in the closure of abdominal wounds versus closure with skin staples in patients undergoing elective colectomy. Int J Colorectal Dis 2010;25:899–905.

40. Romero P, Frongia G, Wingerter S, et al. Prospective, randomized, controlled trial comparing a tissue adhesive (Dermabond) with adhesive strips (Steri-Strips) for the closure of laparoscopic trocar wounds in children. Eur J Pediatr Surg 2011;21:159–62.

41. Souza EC, Fitaroni RB, Januzelli DM, et al. Use of 2-octyl cyanoacrylate for skin closure of sternal incisions in cardiac surgery: observations of microbial barrier effects. Curr Med Res Opin 2008;24:151–5.

42. Davis SC, Eaglstein WH, Cazzaniga AL, et al. An octyl-2-cyanoacrylate formulation speeds healing of partial-thickness wounds. Dermatol Surg 2001;27:783–8.

43. Mertz PM, Davis SC, Cazzaniga AL, et al. Barrier and antibacterial properties of 2-octyl cyanoacrylate-derived wound treatment films. J Cutan Med Surg 2003;7:1–6.

44. Mertz PM, Marshall DA, Eaglstein WH. Occlusive wound dressings to prevent bacterial invasion and wound infection. J Am Acad Dermatol 1985;12:662–8.

45. Moyer CA, Brentano L, Gravens DL, et al. Treatment of large human burns with 0.5 percent silver nitrate solution. Arch Surg 1965;90:812–67.

46. Burrell RE. A scientific perspective on the use of topical silver preparations. Ostomy Wound Manage 2003;49:19–24.

47. Paddle-Ledinek JE, Nasa Z, Cleland HJ. Effect of different wound dressings on cell viability and pro-liferation. Plast Reconstr Surg 2006;117:110S–8S [discussion: 119S–20S].

48. Kostenko V, Lyczak J, Turner K, et al. Impact of silver-containing wound dressings on bacterial bio-film viability and susceptibility to antibiotics during prolonged treatment. Antimicrob Agents Chemother 2010;54:5120–31.

49. Percival SL, Slone W, Linton S, et al. Use of flow cy-tometry to compare the antimicrobial efficacy of silver-containing wound dressings against plank-tonic Staphylococcus aureus and Pseudomonas aeruginosa. Wound Repair Regen 2011;19:436–41.

50. Percival SL, Slone W, Linton S, et al. The antimicro-bial efficacy of a silver alginate dressing against a broad spectrum of clinically relevant wound isolates. Int Wound J 2011;8:237–43.

51. Khundkar R, Malic C, Burge T. Use of Acticoat dressings in burns: what is the evidence? Burns 2010;36:751–8.

52. Caruso DM, Foster KN, Blome-Eberwein SA, et al. Randomized clinical study of hydrofiber dressing with silver or silver sulfadiazine in the management of partial-thickness burns. J Burn Care Res 2006; 27:298–309.

53. Muangman P, Pundee C, Opasanon S, et al. A prospective, randomized trial of silver containing hydrofiber dressing versus 1% silver sulfadiazine for the treatment of partial thickness burns. Int Wound J 2010;7:271–6.

54. Morykwas MJ, Simpson J, Punger K, et al. Vacuum-assisted closure: state of basic research and physi-ologic foundation. Plast Reconstr Surg 2006;117: 121S–6S.

55. Chen SZ, Li J, Li XY, et al. Effects of vacuum-assisted closure on wound microcirculation: an experimental study. Asian J Surg 2005;28:211–7.

56. Wilhelmi BJ, Blackwell SJ, Mancoll JS, et al. Creep vs stretch: a review of the viscoelastic properties of skin. Ann Plast Surg 1998;41:215–9.

57. Chen KD, Li YS, Kim M, et al. Mechanotransduction in response to shear stress. Roles of receptor tyro-sine kinases, integrins, and Shc. J Biol Chem 1999;274:18393–400.

58. Morykwas MJ, Argenta LC, Shelton-Brown EI, et al. Vacuum-assisted closure: a new method for wound control and treatment: animal studies and basic foundation. Ann Plast Surg 1997;38:553–62.

59. Moues CM, Vos MC, van den Bemd GJ, et al. Bacte-rial load in relation to vacuum-assisted closure wound therapy: a prospective randomized trial. Wound Repair Regen 2004;12:11–7.

60. Weed T, Ratliff C, Drake DB. Quantifying bacterial bioburden during negative pressure wound therapy: does the wound VAC enhance bacterial clearance? Ann Plast Surg 2004;52:276–9 [discussion: 279–80].

61. Uygur F, Duman H, Ulkur E, et al. The role of the vacuum-assisted closure therapy in the salvage of venous congestion of the free flap: case report. Int Wound J 2008;5:50–3.

62. Morykwas MJ, Howell H, Bleyer AJ, et al. The effect of externally applied subatmospheric pressure on serum myoglobin levels after a prolonged crush/ischemia injury. J Trauma 2002;53:537–40.

63. Genecov DG, Schneider AM, Morykwas MJ, et al. A controlled subatmospheric pressure dressing increases the rate of skin graft donor site re-epithe-lialization. Ann Plast Surg 1998;40:219–25.

64. Molnar JA, Simpson JL, Voignier DM, et al. Manage-ment of an acute thermal injury with subatmospheric pressure. J Burns Wounds 2005;4:e5.

65. Peinemann F, Sauerland S. Negative-pressure wound therapy: systematic review of randomized controlled trials. Dtsch Arztebl Int 2011;108:381–9.

66. Mikhaylova A, Liesenfeld B, Moore D, et al. Preclin-ical evaluation of antimicrobial efficacy and biocom-patibility of a novel bacterial barrier dressing. Wounds 2011;23:24–31.

67. Youngblood L, Nappo R, JP, et al. Gauze bandages with a bound antimicrobial polymer supress bacte-rial growth in patients with heavily exudating wounds Presented at Symposium on Advanced Wound Care. Dallas (TX), April 14–17, 2011.

Harnessing Growth Factors to Influence Wound Healing

Elizabeth Kiwanuka, MD, Johan Junker, PhD,
Elof Eriksson, MD, PhD*

KEYWORDS

- Cytokines • Growth factors • Wound healing • Gene therapy

KEY POINTS

- The Food and Drug Administration has approved the use of recombinant platelet-derived growth factor for the treatment of lower extremity diabetic neuropathic ulcers that extend into the subcutaneous tissue or beyond and have adequate blood supply.
- Fibroblast growth factor 2, granulocyte-macrophage colony-stimulating factor, and vascular endothelial growth factor are the most promising cytokines and growth factors for the enhancement of wound healing.
- Debridement is the most important step in the treatment of chronic wounds.

INTRODUCTION

The body's response to skin injury is focused on[1–4]:

1. Rapid wound closure
2. Restraining invasion of microorganisms
3. Preventing excessive fluid loss.

The early response is activated immediately after injury, resulting in the inflammatory phase (first stage) of wound healing.[5] After hemostasis a fibrin clot is formed, which later serves as a scaffold for infiltrating cells. In addition, neutrophils and monocytes are recruited to the wound in response to trauma and bacterial contamination.[6]

The second stage of wound repair occurs approximately 2 to 10 days after the injury and is characterized by proliferation and migration of different cell types. Keratinocytes migrate over the wound bed while fibroblasts and macrophages replace the fibrin clot with granulation tissue.[7] The newly formed immature dermis is neovascularized, and the keratinocytes behind the leading edge proliferate and differentiate to restore the barrier function of the epidermis.

Tissue remodeling, the third stage of wound repair, begins 2 to 3 weeks after injury and lasts for 1 year or more. The type III collagen that is deposited in the initial stages of wound healing is slowly replaced by type I collagen, thereby forming the mature dermis.[8]

An increased understanding of the molecular mechanisms that regulate the various events of wound healing has laid the foundation for therapeutic interventions attempting to improve the healing outcome. The cell-cell and cell-matrix interactions are fundamental for successful wound healing, and growth factors and cytokines maintain the balance of signals that regulate cellular migration, proliferation, and adhesion to a large extent.[9–12] Malfunction leads to a prolonged healing time or complete failure to heal and may result in a chronic wound. The wound fluid from chronic wounds has an increased concentration of proinflammatory cytokines in comparison with wound fluid from acute wounds.[13,14] By contrast, there

Division of Plastic Surgery, Brigham and Women's Hospital, Harvard Medical School, 75 Francis Street, Boston, MA 02115, USA
* Corresponding author.
E-mail address: eeriksson@partners.org

Clin Plastic Surg 39 (2012) 239–248
doi:10.1016/j.cps.2012.04.003

is a decreased concentration of growth factors in chronic wounds with high protease activity and decreased levels of natural protease inhibitors.[15–17] This deficiency in growth factors can be attributable to decreased production or secretion, more rapid breakdown, and, as is the case in venous stasis ulcers, binding to macromolecules, making them nonfunctional.[14,18]

CYTOKINES AND GROWTH FACTORS IN WOUND HEALING
Cytokines in Wound Healing

Cytokines are peptides and glycoproteins with a molecular weight of 5 to 30 kDa and are primarily produced by inflammatory cells.[19] Cytokines regulate inflammatory and immune responses during wound healing by activating various cells. The cytokines include chemokines, lymphokines, monokines, interleukins, colony-stimulating factors, and interferons, and can be distinguished from growth factors by the type of cells they influence. Inflammatory cytokines are believed to have roles in wound healing, including migration and proliferation of keratinocytes and fibroblasts.[20] Interleukins 1 and 6 (IL-1 and IL-6) and tumor necrosis factor α (TNF-α) are upregulated during the inflammatory phase of wound healing and are important in modulating reepithelialization.[11] The granulocyte-macrophage colony-stimulating factor (GM-CSF) is involved in the activation of neutrophils and macrophages, and alters the activity of keratinocytes and fibroblasts.[21]

Interleukins in Wound Healing

In an acute wound, IL-1 is produced by monocytes, macrophages, fibroblasts, and keratinocytes.[22–24] Besides serving as a paracrine factor, IL-1 acts as an autocrine signal that induces the migration and proliferation of keratinocytes.[9,25,26] Exogenously administered IL-1 has been shown to promote healing of partial-thickness wounds in swine.[27] In a prospective, double-blind, placebo-controlled trial, various concentrations of IL-1β were administered to patients with pressure ulcers daily for 28 days.[28] No significant differences were noted in any of the treatment groups.

TNF-α in Wound Healing

Similar to IL-1, TNF-α is a proinflammatory cytokine that is produced by many cell types during wound healing.[29] The TNF-α level is elevated in chronic wounds, and its expression diminishes as healing progresses. In a study by Streit and colleagues,[30] the TNF-α antagonist infliximab was administered daily to 14 leg ulcers. After 4 weeks of treatment, the surface area of the ulcer was reduced by more than 50% in 6 of the 14 leg ulcers.

GM-CSF

GM-CSF is one of the most widely studied cytokines in wound healing.[21,31,32] Besides being a potent activator of neutrophils and macrophages, GM-CSF influences the activity of keratinocytes and fibroblasts and increases the production of vascular endothelial growth factor (VEGF).[33] In a double-blind, randomized, controlled study of 60 patients with venous stasis ulcers, GM-CSF was perilesionally injected weekly for 4 weeks. Administration of GM-CSF significantly improved the rate of healing by approximately 60%.[34]

Growth Factors in Wound Healing

Growth factors are regulatory peptides that are synthesized and secreted by many of the cell types involved in wound healing, including inflammatory cells, platelets, fibroblasts, epithelial cells, and endothelial cells.[35] Growth factors cause cells to migrate by chemotaxis, proliferate, differentiate, and synthesize extracellular matrix components.[36] Growth factors may act by autocrine, paracrine, juxtacrine, or endocrine signaling. On binding to the cell receptors, the growth factors trigger a cascade of intracellular events, leading to the activation of transcription factors, which results in gene expression.

Growth factors are classified into several families based on their characteristics. The most relevant growth factor families for wound healing are the epidermal growth factor (EGF), fibroblast growth factor (FGF), transforming growth factor β (TGF-β), platelet-derived growth factor (PDGF), and VEGF. The different growth factor families are summarized in **Table 1**.

EGF family
The EGF family consists of:

- EGF
- TGF-α
- Amphiregulin
- Heparin-binding EGF.

EGF was first isolated from the submandibular glands of rats but is primarily produced by platelets and macrophages.[37] The roles of the EGFs and growth factors that signal through the EGF receptor (EGFR) are well characterized. The EGFR is a transmembrane protein tyrosine kinase that is expressed on many different cell types.[38] Numerous in vitro studies have shown that activation of the EGFR increases the migration[39,40] and

Table 1
Cytokines and growth factors in wound healing

	Cells	Effects During Wound Healing
Cytokine		
IL-1	Neutrophils Monocytes Macrophages Keratinocytes	Inflammation, reepithelialization, increased levels in the acute and chronic wound
Growth Factors		
EGF	Platelets Macrophages Fibroblasts	Cell motility and proliferation, increased levels in the acute wound, decreased levels in the chronic wound
TGF-β1 and TGF-β2	Platelets Keratinocytes Macrophages Lymphocytes Fibroblasts	Reepithelialization and inflammation, granulation tissue formation, fibrosis and tensile strength, increased levels in the acute wound, decreased levels in the chronic wound
PDGF	Platelets Keratinocytes Macrophages Endothelial cells Fibroblasts	Chemotaxis, inflammation, granulation tissue formation, matrix remodeling, increased levels in the acute wound, decreased levels in the chronic wound
VEGF	Platelets Neutrophils Macrophages Endothelial cells Fibroblasts	Angiogenesis, granulation tissue formation, increased levels in the acute wound, decreased levels in the chronic wound
IL-1	Neutrophils Monocytes Macrophages Keratinocytes	Inflammation, reepithelialization, increased levels in the acute and chronic wound

proliferation[41,42] of keratinocytes. However, in vivo wound-healing studies using knockout mice have generated conflicting results. Abnormal epidermal proliferation has been noted in EGFR-null skin grafts that have been transplanted to nude mice.[43] Early studies using TGF-α–deficient mice showed no decrease in the rate of reepithelialization,[44,45] whereas later studies found that partial-thickness wounds in mice exhibited a decrease in the rate of reepithelialization.[46]

Although there is an agreement that addition of exogenous EGFR ligand improves wound closure by increasing reepithelialization, it is not clear whether the extent of improvement is of such clinical significance to warrant the use of EGF ligands as therapeutic agents. In 1989, Brown and colleagues[47] performed the first clinical trial in which a recombinant growth factor was added to accelerate wound healing. Partial-thickness skin graft donor sites in patients with burns were treated with EGFs in Silvadene cream (1% silver sulfadiazine) and compared with paired control sites treated with Silvadene cream alone. The EGF-treated wounds reached 25% and 50% healing by an average of 1 day earlier than the control wounds, and the time to 100% healing was reduced by an average of 1.5 days. Although the EGF-treated group experienced a better healing outcome based on a higher level of cellular organization than the control group, the results were not considered clinically significant.

FGF family

The FGF family has more than 20 members, of which the most relevant for wound healing are

- FGF-2
- FGF-7
- FGF-10
- FGF-22

FGF-7 is also known as the keratinocyte growth factor 1 (KGF-1) and is secreted by dermal fibroblasts and T cells.[48–50] FGF-10 is closely homologous to FGF-7 and acts on keratinocytes to increase migration and proliferation.[51] FGF-22 is expressed in an autocrine manner by hair follicle keratinocytes and can be found in the later stages of wound healing.

FGF-2, also known as basic FGF, is released from damaged endothelial cells and is one of the most potent isoforms. FGF-2 is a mitogenic and chemotactic factor for fibroblasts and endothelial cells, and stimulates angiogenesis. Its concentration is upregulated during wound healing, and exogenous administration of FGF-2 has been shown to increase wound reepithelialization.[52,53] In knockout studies, FGF-2–deficient mice have been found to have impaired wound healing.[54,55] Based on in vitro data and preclinical experiments, Robson and colleagues[56] treated 50 patients with pressure ulcers with recombinant FGF-2. After debridement of the wounds, various concentrations of recombinant FGF-2 were topically applied daily for a treatment period of 30 days. There was a trend toward faster healing in the treated wounds than in the controls. In another study, Robson and colleagues[57] treated patients with venous ulcers with topical application of GM-CSF and FGF-2, sequential application of GM-CSF and FGF-1, or vehicle placebo in a double-blinded randomized manner. The patients received daily treatments for 35 days, whereas the sequential group received GM-CSF for 10 days and FGF-2 for 25 days. The results showed that treatment with GM-CSF and/or FGF-2 resulted in improved healing as well as increased levels of PDGF, FGF-2, and TGF-β1 in the wound tissue. In another study, FGF-2 was topically applied daily for 6 weeks and then twice a week for 12 weeks to 17 patients with diabetic foot ulcers in a double-blinded, randomized manner.[58] No significant difference was observed.

TGF-β family

The TGF-β family consists of[59]

- TGF-β1–3
- Bone morphogenetic proteins (BMPs)
- Activins
- Nodals
- Growth and differentiation factors
- Mullerian-inhibiting substances.

The TGF-β superfamily is so named because it was believed to induce normal cells to become malignant.[60] At present, TGF-β cells are seen as important regulators of wound healing. Clinical studies have primarily focused on the 3 isoforms of TGF-β and the BMPs. TGF-β1 and TGF-β2 are secreted by several different cell types and have overall profibrotic effects, with increased formation of granulation tissue and stimulation of wound contraction. TGF-β1 and TGF-β2 increase the synthesis of matrix components, such as collagen and fibronectin, and inhibit the synthesis of matrix-degrading enzymes. TGF-β3, on the other hand, may have greater anti-inflammatory properties.[61]

The role of TGF-β in wound healing is not fully understood. TGF-β has been shown to inhibit keratinocyte proliferation both in vitro and in vivo.[62–64] However, other studies have shown that overexpression of TGF-β1 increases the proliferative phenotype of the epidermis.[65,66] Exogenous TGF-β has been shown to increase keratinocyte migration in vitro, and these results are in concordance with a study showing increased migration of keratinocytes in partial-thickness porcine skin explants after the addition of TGF-β.[66] TGF-β antagonists have been shown to increase reepithelialization of full-thickness wounds in pigs.[67]

Role of TGF-β in ulcer studies In a prospective, randomized, double-blinded, placebo-controlled study, venous stasis ulcers were treated with TGF-β2.[68] The TGF-β2 was administered using a lyophilized collagen sponge and the results were compared with those in patients treated with TGF-β2 using a sponge alone or wound dressing. Ulcers treated with TGF-β2 showed a 57% decrease in size, whereas those treated with sponge alone or dressing showed a decrease of 30% and 9%, respectively.

TGF-β3 was evaluated in a randomized, double-blinded, placebo-controlled study involving 14 patients with pressure ulcers who received TGF-β3 or placebo in various concentrations.[69] TGF-β3 was sprayed onto the wound bed using a syringe, and wounds were treated daily for 16 weeks or until complete healing. Wounds treated with TGF-β3 demonstrated increased healing at 4 weeks in comparison with the controls, but there were no significant differences at the end of the study.

Role of TGF-β in bone studies Of the BMPs, BMP-1 and BMP-7 have been generated in a recombinant form suitable for clinical applications.[70] The BMPs have primarily been used to heal fractures.[71,72] After its efficacy was demonstrated, recombinant BMP-2 has been approved for human use in the treatment of lumbar fusion, and recombinant BMP-7 has been approved by the US Food and Drug Administration (FDA) for clinical use in the healing of the spine.

PDGF family

The PDGF is the first and only recombinant growth factor to be approved by the FDA for topical administration to wounds. The PDGF family consists of several homodimeric or heterodimeric growth factors including

- PDGF-AA
- PDGF-BB
- PDGF-AB.

PDGF is produced by

- Platelets
- Macrophages
- Endothelial cells
- Fibroblasts
- Keratinocytes.

Each of these cells plays a role in each phase of wound healing.[73,74]

PDGF-BB accelerates the formation of granulation tissue to a greater extent than PDGF-AA both in vitro and in vivo.[75] PDGF increases collagen production by fibroblasts and induces a myofibroblastic phenotype. In addition, PDGF promotes angiogenesis by stimulating endothelial migration. PDGF is released from platelets on injury and can be found in the wound fluid in acute wounds.[76] By contrast, PDGF levels are less in the wound fluid of chronic wounds.[77]

The role of PDGF in diabetic foot ulcers PDGF-BB has successfully been administered to diabetic foot ulcers to enhance wound healing. In a double-blind, placebo-controlled, multicenter study, 118 patients with chronic full-thickness diabetic neuropathic ulcers were treated with recombinant human PDGF-BB or placebo for 20 weeks or until complete healing.[78] Of the 61 patients who were treated with recombinant human PDGF-BB, 48% achieved complete wound healing compared with 25% of the 57 patients treated with placebo. This was the significant difference that led the FDA to approve recombinant human PDGF-BB in a preparation called becaplermin. The preparation is sold by Johnson & Johnson Wound Management under the trade name Regranex.

VEGF family
The members of the VEGF family include

- VEGF-A
- VEGF-B
- VEGF-C
- VEGF-D
- VEGF-E
- Placental growth factor.

The VEGF is produced by a variety of cell types during wound healing, and is a potent stimulator of proliferation and migration in endothelial cells.[79,80]

Increased expression of VEGF-A is seen in ischemic wounds as well as in several chronic wounds, which have areas of local skin ischemia, therefore making VEGF-A a possible therapeutic modality.[81] Administration of VEGF-A improved impaired angiogenesis in the ischemic limbs of patients with diabetes. Other in vivo experiments show that VEGF-A enhances reepithelialization of diabetic wounds by increasing vessel formation.[82] Although VEGF has been shown to promote healing in various experimental models, there is no recombinant VEGF available for topical application. Antibodies targeting soluble VEGF are currently being used in anticancer therapies.[83] **Table 1** summarizes the cytokines and growth factors in wound healing.

TOPICAL APPLICATION OF GROWTH FACTORS AND WOUND HEALING

Normally the skin is a barrier against mechanical and chemical insults, and the epidermis particularly provides a substantial barrier to the topical application of drugs and therapeutics. However, on cutaneous injury the epidermal barrier is disrupted, which facilitates administration of cytokines and growth factors to the wound bed.

Several studies have been performed on the effect of topically applied factors in experimental wound healing since the development of recombinant growth factors.[84] Clinically source data exist for chronic wounds, and cytokines and growth factors have been administered as a single agent, in combinations, or sequentially. The effects of recombinant peptide growth factors were initially promising, but direct application of peptide factors to the wound environment carries several limitations. The half-life is generally short, necessitating repeated administration. The growth factors are susceptible to degradation by the abundant proteolytic enzymes in the wound environment. Furthermore, sequestration of growth factors by the wound matrix may hinder its binding to receptors at the surfaces of the cells. Improved delivery systems or carriers will have to be developed for recombinant growth factors to become an attractive option in wound therapy.[85]

GENE THERAPY FOR WOUND HEALING

As the body's largest and most accessible organ, the skin is an attractive target for gene therapy. The skin is easy to access, allowing the direct transfer of DNA and RNA through several techniques, including injection, microseeding, electroporation, and topical application. Systemic delivery can be reduced using these techniques. Fibroblasts and keratinocytes can be easily harvested and cultured, allowing gene transfer in vitro. The superficial location of the skin enables repeated monitoring of the effects of the therapy. Prolonged gene expression is limited by the high turnover time of the epidermis, which reduces the risks of long-term side effects.[86]

Gene therapy offers several advantages over the direct administration of peptide factors:

- Peptides delivered to the wound environment are highly susceptible to proteolytic degradation, thereby lowering the effective dose.
- Sequestration by the wound matrix may prevent the binding to receptors at the surfaces of the cells.
- Gene therapy allows the sustained and regulated secretion of factors in their proper spatial and temporal contexts. This aspect is particularly important, as growth factors may have different effects depending on cell type, concentration, and other simultaneous signals from soluble factors, adhesion molecules, and matrix components.

A wide range of gene-therapy approaches has been used for wounds in the experimental setting. Growth factor genes have been widely used in experimental gene therapy to enhance wound healing. The most commonly used approach has been to overexpress genes that stimulate reepithelialization, angiogenesis, or fibroplasia. Various methods have been deployed for gene delivery. Furthermore, transgene-containing vectors have been directly applied to wounds for in situ transformation or used in vitro in approaches based on cell therapy. An emerging concept is the use of biomaterial scaffolds as carriers of in vitro transformed cells and growth factors to the site of tissue repair.[87]

In the ischemic rat ear model, the delivery of PDGF-B to wounds was mediated by adenoviral vectors.[88] The wounds to which PDGF-B was administered showed an increase in the rate of reepithelialization in comparison with control wounds. However, the adenoviral particles themselves impaired wound healing, presumably because of an increased local inflammatory response. Adenoviral delivery of PDGF-B was used in the first clinical trial of gene therapy in wound healing, which demonstrated that periulcer injection with a replication-incompetent vector was well tolerated and improved wound healing.[89] It appeared that the overexpression of PDGF-B enhanced vasculogenesis, and the investigators

concluded that the protocol should be considered for further studies in humans.

Several investigators have used gene therapy with VEGF to enhance healing in diabetic as well as nondiabetic rodent models.[90–93] Other growth factors that are adenovirally delivered in animal wound models are TGF-β, placental growth factor, and KGF.[94–96] The signaling of growth factors may also be inhibited by gene therapy. The truncated TGF-β receptor II, delivered to a rodent wound model by adenoviral vectors, inhibited TGF-β signaling, inflammation, and scar formation.[97]

Since the 1990s, RNA interference has become a major subject of interest as a therapeutic approach for gene-related diseases. ALN-RSV01 is the first example of an antiviral small interfering RNA (siRNA)-based therapeutic targeting the human respiratory syncytial virus after viral infection, and the first example of an antivirus siRNA-based therapeutic in a phase I clinical study. The use of siRNAs for the sequence-specific knockdown of disease-causing genes has led to numerous preclinical studies.[98,99]

FUTURE PERSPECTIVES ON GROWTH FACTORS FOR WOUND HEALING

Cytokines and growth factors have been administered using various approaches in an attempt to optimize the molecular environment in the healing wound. These agents have become available for clinical use since the development of the recombinant technology. The topical administration of cytokines and growth factors to chronic wounds exposes recombinant peptides to proteolytic enzymes and, therefore, repeated administrations are often required. Some of these hurdles can be overcome by the use of alternative administrations, such as gene therapy. In addition, new delivery systems, such as scaffolds and slow-releasing polymers, are being investigated as delivery systems for cytokines and growth factors.

FGF-2, GM-CSF, and VEGF are the most promising cytokines and growth factors for the enhancement of wound healing. Further clinical studies are required to elucidate the efficiency and safety of such treatment additions in wound healing. At present, recombinant PDGF-BB is used in the treatment of lower extremity diabetic neuropathic ulcers that extend into the subcutaneous tissue or beyond and have adequate blood supply. Studies to assess the use of recombinant PDGF-BB in the treatment of other types of chronic wounds are under way.

Although several methods of delivering cytokines and growth factors to the healing wound are available, the use of peptides in wound healing remains limited. In the healing wound, several cytokines and growth factors act in concert, and the complicated patterns of expression are not completely understood.

SUMMARY

Manipulating the microenvironment of the healing wound by the addition of growth factors and cytokines has been attempted, with promising results. A better understanding of the cellular and molecular events that occur during wound healing needs to be gained to further optimize the scheme of delivery. The optimization and development of current delivery methods will also improve the utility of growth factors for the treatment of wounds.

REFERENCES

1. Singer AJ, Clark RA. Cutaneous wound healing. N Engl J Med 1999;341:738–46.
2. Aarabi S, Longaker MT, Gurtner GC. Hypertrophic scar formation following burns and trauma: new approaches to treatment. PLoS Med 2007;4:e234.
3. Gurtner GC, Werner S, Barrandon Y, et al. Wound repair and regeneration. Nature 2008;453:314–21.
4. Mustoe T. Understanding chronic wounds: a unifying hypothesis on their pathogenesis and implications for therapy. Am J Surg 2004;187:65S–70S.
5. Grose R, Werner S. Wound-healing studies in transgenic and knockout mice. Mol Biotechnol 2004;28:147–66.
6. Martin P, Leibovich SJ. Inflammatory cells during wound repair: the good, the bad and the ugly. Trends Cell Biol 2005;15:599–607.
7. Werner S, Krieg T, Smola H. Keratinocyte-fibroblast interactions in wound healing. J Invest Dermatol 2007;127:998–1008.
8. Lovvorn HN 3rd, Cheung DT, Nimni ME, et al. Relative distribution and crosslinking of collagen distinguish fetal from adult sheep wound repair. J Pediatr Surg 1999;34:218–23.
9. Freedberg IM, Tomic-Canic M, Komine M, et al. Keratins and the keratinocyte activation cycle. J Invest Dermatol 2001;116:633–40.
10. Hantash BM, Zhao L, Knowles JA, et al. Adult and fetal wound healing. Front Biosci 2008;13:51–61.
11. Werner S, Grose R. Regulation of wound healing by growth factors and cytokines. Physiol Rev 2003;83:835–70.
12. Barrientos S, Stojadinovic O, Golinko MS, et al. Growth factors and cytokines in wound healing. Wound Repair Regen 2008;16:585–601.
13. Bennett NT, Schultz GS. Growth factors and wound healing: Part II. Role in normal and chronic wound healing. Am J Surg 1993;166:74–81.
14. Robson MC, Hill DP, Woodske ME, et al. Wound healing trajectories as predictors of effectiveness of therapeutic agents. Arch Surg 2000;135:773–7.
15. Nwomeh BC, Yager DR, Cohen IK. Physiology of the chronic wound. Clin Plast Surg 1998;25:341–56.
16. Mast BA, Schultz GS. Interactions of cytokines, growth factors, and proteases in acute and chronic wounds. Wound Repair Regen 1996;4:411–20.
17. Tarnuzzer RW, Schultz GS. Biochemical analysis of acute and chronic wound environments. Wound Repair Regen 1996;4:321–5.
18. Falanga V, Eaglstein WH. The "trap" hypothesis of venous ulceration. Lancet 1993;341:1006–8.
19. Rumalla VK, Borah GL. Cytokines, growth factors, and plastic surgery. Plast Reconstr Surg 2001;108:719–33.
20. Holman DM, Kalaaji AN. Cytokines in dermatology. J Drugs Dermatol 2006;5:520–4.
21. Hu X, Sun H, Han C, et al. Topically applied rhGM-CSF for the wound healing: a systematic review. Burns 2011;37:729–41.
22. Sauder DN, Kilian PL, McLane JA, et al. Interleukin-1 enhances epidermal wound healing. Lymphokine Res 1990;9:465–73.
23. Goretsky MJ, Harriger MD, Supp AP, et al. Expression of interleukin-1alpha, interleukin-6, and basic fibroblast growth factor by cultured skin substitutes before and after grafting to full-thickness wounds in athymic mice. J Trauma 1996;40:894–9 [discussion: 899–900].
24. Finnerty CC, Herndon DN, Przkora R, et al. Cytokine expression profile over time in severely burned pediatric patients. Shock 2006;26:13–9.
25. Chen JD, Lapiere JC, Sauder DN, et al. Interleukin-1 alpha stimulates keratinocyte migration through an epidermal growth factor/transforming growth factor-alpha-independent pathway. J Invest Dermatol 1995;104:729–33.
26. Gyulai R, Hunyadi J, Kenderessy-Szabo A, et al. Chemotaxis of freshly separated and cultured human keratinocytes. Clin Exp Dermatol 1994;19:309–11.
27. Singer AJ, McClain SA, Hacht G, et al. Semapimod reduces the depth of injury resulting in enhanced re-epithelialization of partial-thickness burns in swine. J Burn Care Res 2006;27:40–9.
28. Robson MC, Abdullah A, Burns BF, et al. Safety and effect of topical recombinant human interleukin-1beta in the management of pressure sores. Wound Repair Regen 1994;2:177–81.
29. Brauchle M, Angermeyer K, Hubner G, et al. Large induction of keratinocyte growth factor expression by serum growth factors and pro-inflammatory cytokines in cultured fibroblasts. Oncogene 1994;9:3199–204.
30. Streit M, Beleznay Z, Braathen LR. Topical application of the tumour necrosis factor-alpha antibody

infliximab improves healing of chronic wounds. Int Wound J 2006;3:171–9.

31. Malik IA, Zahid M, Haq S, et al. Effect of subcutaneous injection of granulocyte-macrophage colony stimulating factor (GM-CSF) on healing of chronic refractory wounds. Eur J Surg 1998;164:737–44.

32. Jaschke E, Zabernigg A, Gattringer C. Recombinant human granulocyte-macrophage colony-stimulating factor applied locally in low doses enhances healing and prevents recurrence of chronic venous ulcers. Int J Dermatol 1999;38:380–6.

33. Cruciani M, Lipsky BA, Mengoli C, et al. Are granulocyte colony-stimulating factors beneficial in treating diabetic foot infections?: a meta-analysis. Diabetes Care 2005;28:454–60.

34. Da Costa RM, Ribeiro Jesus FM, Aniceto C, et al. Randomized, double-blind, placebo-controlled, dose-ranging study of granulocyte-macrophage colony stimulating factor in patients with chronic venous leg ulcers. Wound Repair Regen 1999;7:17–25.

35. Bennett NT, Schultz GS. Growth factors and wound healing: biochemical properties of growth factors and their receptors. Am J Surg 1993;165:728–37.

36. Robson MC. Growth factors as wound healing agents. Curr Opin Biotechnol 1991;2:863–7.

37. Cohen S. Isolation of a mouse submaxillary gland protein accelerating incisor eruption and eyelid opening in the new-born animal. J Biol Chem 1962;237:1555–62.

38. Yarden Y. The EGFR family and its ligands in human cancer. Signalling mechanisms and therapeutic opportunities. Eur J Cancer 2001;37(Suppl 4):S3–8.

39. Cha D, O'Brien P, O'Toole EA, et al. Enhanced modulation of keratinocyte motility by transforming growth factor-alpha (TGF-alpha) relative to epidermal growth factor (EGF). J Invest Dermatol 1996;106:590–7.

40. McCawley LJ, O'Brien P, Hudson LG. Epidermal growth factor (EGF)- and scatter factor/hepatocyte growth factor (SF/HGF)-mediated keratinocyte migration is coincident with induction of matrix metalloproteinase (MMP)-9. J Cell Physiol 1998;176:255–65.

41. Martin P. Wound healing—aiming for perfect skin regeneration. Science 1997;276:75–81.

42. Rheinwald JG, Green H. Epidermal growth factor and the multiplication of cultured human epidermal keratinocytes. Nature 1977;265:421–4.

43. Haase I, Evans R, Pofahl R, et al. Regulation of keratinocyte shape, migration and wound epithelialization by IGF-1- and EGF-dependent signalling pathways. J Cell Sci 2003;116:3227–38.

44. Luetteke NC, Qiu TH, Peiffer RL, et al. TGF alpha deficiency results in hair follicle and eye abnormalities in targeted and waved-1 mice. Cell 1993;73:263–78.

45. Mann GB, Fowler KJ, Gabriel A, et al. Mice with a null mutation of the TGF alpha gene have abnormal skin architecture, wavy hair, and curly whiskers and often develop corneal inflammation. Cell 1993;73:249–61.

46. Kim I, Mogford JE, Chao JD, et al. Wound epithelialization deficits in the transforming growth factor-alpha knockout mouse. Wound Repair Regen 2001;9:386–90.

47. Brown GL, Nanney LB, Griffen J, et al. Enhancement of wound healing by topical treatment with epidermal growth factor. N Engl J Med 1989;321:76–9.

48. Jameson J, Ugarte K, Chen N, et al. A role for skin gammadelta T cells in wound repair. Science 2002;296:747–9.

49. auf demKeller U, Krampert M, Kumin A, et al. Keratinocyte growth factor: effects on keratinocytes and mechanisms of action. Eur J Cell Biol 2004;83:607–12.

50. Steiling H, Werner S. Fibroblast growth factors: key players in epithelial morphogenesis, repair and cytoprotection. Curr Opin Biotechnol 2003;14:533–7.

51. Igarashi M, Finch PW, Aaronson SA. Characterization of recombinant human fibroblast growth factor (FGF)-10 reveals functional similarities with keratinocyte growth factor (FGF-7). J Biol Chem 1998;273:13230–5.

52. Sanz Garcia S, Santos Heredero X, Izquierdo Hernandez A, et al. Experimental model for local application of growth factors in skin re-epithelialisation. Scand J Plast Reconstr Surg Hand Surg 2000;34:199–206.

53. Hebda PA, Klingbeil CK, Abraham JA, et al. Basic fibroblast growth factor stimulation of epidermal wound healing in pigs. J Invest Dermatol 1990;95:626–31.

54. Marchese C, Chedid M, Dirsch OR, et al. Modulation of keratinocyte growth factor and its receptor in ree-pithelializing human skin. J Exp Med 1995;182:1369–76.

55. Ortega S, Ittmann M, Tsang SH, et al. Neuronal defects and delayed wound healing in mice lacking fibroblast growth factor 2. Proc Natl Acad Sci U S A 1998;95:5672–7.

56. Robson MC, Phillips LG, Lawrence WT, et al. The safety and effect of topically applied recombinant basic fibroblast growth factor on the healing of chronic pressure sores. Ann Surg 1992;216:401–6 [discussion: 406–8].

57. Robson MC, Hill DP, Smith PD, et al. Sequential cytokine therapy for pressure ulcers: clinical and mechanistic response. Ann Surg 2000;231:600–11.

58. Richard JL, Parer-Richard C, Daures JP, et al. Effect of topical basic fibroblast growth factor on the healing of chronic diabetic neuropathic ulcer of the foot.

A pilot, randomized, double-blind, placebo-controlled study. Diabetes Care 1995;18:64–9.

59. Shi Y, Massague J. Mechanisms of TGF-beta signaling from cell membrane to the nucleus. Cell 2003;113:685–700.

60. Broughton G 2nd, Janis JE, Attinger CE. The basic science of wound healing. Plast Reconstr Surg 2006;117:12S–34S.

61. Douglas HE. TGF-β in wound healing: a review. J Wound Care 2010;19:403–6.

62. Coffey RJ Jr, Bascom CC, Sipes NJ, et al. Selective inhibition of growth-related gene expression in murine keratinocytes by transforming growth factor beta. Mol Cell Biol 1988;8:3088–93.

63. Sellheyer K, Bickenbach JR, Rothnagel JA, et al. Inhibition of skin development by overexpression of transforming growth factor beta 1 in the epidermis of transgenic mice. Proc Natl Acad Sci U S A 1993; 90:5237–41.

64. Yang L, Chan T, Demare J, et al. Healing of burn wounds in transgenic mice overexpressing transforming growth factor-beta 1 in the epidermis. Am J Pathol 2001;159:2147–57.

65. Ito Y, Sarkar P, Mi Q, et al. Overexpression of Smad2 reveals its concerted action with Smad4 in regulating TGF-beta-mediated epidermal homeostasis. Dev Biol 2001;236:181–94.

66. Li AG, Wang D, Feng XH, et al. Latent TGFbeta1 overexpression in keratinocytes results in a severe psoriasis-like skin disorder. EMBO J 2004;23: 1770–81.

67. Huang JS, Wang YH, Ling TY, et al. Synthetic TGF-beta antagonist accelerates wound healing and reduces scarring. FASEB J 2002;16:1269–70.

68. Robson MC, Phillip LG, Cooper DM, et al. Safety and effect of transforming growth factor-beta(2) for treatment of venous stasis ulcers. Wound Repair Regen 1995;3:157–67.

69. Hirshberg J, Coleman J, Marchant B, et al. TGF-beta3 in the treatment of pressure ulcers: a preliminary report. Adv Skin Wound Care 2001;14: 91–5.

70. Cheng H, Jiang W, Phillips FM, et al. Osteogenic activity of the fourteen types of human bone morphogenetic proteins (BMPs). J Bone Joint Surg Am 2003;85:1544–52.

71. Burkus JK, Transfeldt EE, Kitchel SH, et al. Clinical and radiographic outcomes of anterior lumbar interbody fusion using recombinant human bone morphogenetic protein-2. Spine (Phila Pa 1976) 2002;27:2396–408.

72. Govender S, Csimma C, Genant HK, et al. Recombinant human bone morphogenetic protein-2 for treatment of open tibial fractures: a prospective, controlled, randomized study of four hundred and fifty patients. J Bone Joint Surg Am 2002;84: 2123–34.

73. Niessen FB, Andriessen MP, Schalkwijk J, et al. Keratinocyte-derived growth factors play a role in the formation of hypertrophic scars. J Pathol 2001;194: 207–16.

74. Uutela M, Wirzenius M, Paavonen K, et al. PDGF-D induces macrophage recruitment, increased interstitial pressure, and blood vessel maturation during angiogenesis. Blood 2004;104:3198–204.

75. Bennett SP, Griffiths GD, Schor AM, et al. Growth factors in the treatment of diabetic foot ulcers. Br J Surg 2003;90:133–46.

76. Vogt PM, Lehnhardt M, Wagner D, et al. Determination of endogenous growth factors in human wound fluid: temporal presence and profiles of secretion. Plast Reconstr Surg 1998;102:117–23.

77. Trengove NJ, Bielefeldt-Ohmann H, Stacey MC. Mitogenic activity and cytokine levels in non-healing and healing chronic leg ulcers. Wound Repair Regen 2000;8:13–25.

78. Steed DL. Clinical evaluation of recombinant human platelet-derived growth factor for the treatment of lower extremity diabetic ulcers. Diabetic Ulcer Study Group. J Vasc Surg 1995;21:71–8 [discussion: 79–81].

79. Nissen NN, Polverini PJ, Koch AE, et al. Vascular endothelial growth factor mediates angiogenic activity during the proliferative phase of wound healing. Am J Pathol 1998;152:1445–52.

80. Gaudry M, Bregerie O, Andrieu V, et al. Intracellular pool of vascular endothelial growth factor in human neutrophils. Blood 1997;90:4153–61.

81. Pepper MS, Ferrara N, Orci L, et al. Potent synergism between vascular endothelial growth factor and basic fibroblast growth factor in the induction of angiogenesis in vitro. Biochem Biophys Res Commun 1992;189:824–31.

82. Galiano RD, Tepper OM, Pelo CR, et al. Topical vascular endothelial growth factor accelerates diabetic wound healing through increased angiogenesis and by mobilizing and recruiting bone marrow-derived cells. Am J Pathol 2004;164:1935–47.

83. Geva R, Prenen H, Topal B, et al. Biologic modulation of chemotherapy in patients with hepatic colorectal metastases: the role of anti-VEGF and anti-EGFR antibodies. J Surg Oncol 2010;102: 937–45.

84. Pierce GF, Tarpley JE, Tseng J, et al. Detection of platelet-derived growth factor (PDGF)-AA in actively healing human wounds treated with recombinant PDGF-BB and absence of PDGF in chronic nonhealing wounds. J Clin Invest 1995;96:1336–50.

85. Robson MC, Mustoe TA, Hunt TK. The future of recombinant growth factors in wound healing. Am J Surg 1998;176:80S–2S.

86. Bevan S, Martin R, McKay IA. The production and applications of genetically modified skin cells. Biotechnol Genet Eng Rev 1999;16:231–56.

87. Jang JH, Houchin TL, Shea LD. Gene delivery from polymer scaffolds for tissue engineering. Expert Rev Med Devices 2004;1:127–38.

88. Liechty KW, Nesbit M, Herlyn M, et al. Adenoviral-mediated overexpression of platelet-derived growth factor-B corrects ischemic impaired wound healing. J Invest Dermatol 1999;113:375–83.

89. Margolis DJ, Crombleholme T, Herlyn M. Clinical protocol: phase I trial to evaluate the safety of H5.020CMV.PDGF-B for the treatment of a diabetic insensate foot ulcer. Wound Repair Regen 2000;8:480–93.

90. Brem H, Kodra A, Golinko MS, et al. Mechanism of sustained release of vascular endothelial growth factor in accelerating experimental diabetic healing. J Invest Dermatol 2009;129:2275–87.

91. Saaristo A, Tammela T, Farkkila A, et al. Vascular endothelial growth factor-C accelerates diabetic wound healing. Am J Pathol 2006;169:1080–7.

92. Ailawadi M, Lee JM, Lee S, et al. Adenovirus vector-mediated transfer of the vascular endothelial growth factor cDNA to healing abdominal fascia enhances vascularity and bursting strength in mice with normal and impaired wound healing. Surgery 2002;131:219–27.

93. Romano Di Peppe S, Mangoni A, Zambruno G, et al. Adenovirus-mediated VEGF(165) gene transfer enhances wound healing by promoting angiogenesis in CD1 diabetic mice. Gene Ther 2002;9:1271–7.

94. Lee B, Vouthounis C, Stojadinovic O, et al. From an enhanceosome to a repressosome: molecular antagonism between glucocorticoids and EGF leads to inhibition of wound healing. J Mol Biol 2005;345:1083–97.

95. Escamez MJ, Carretero M, Garcia M, et al. Assessment of optimal virus-mediated growth factor gene delivery for human cutaneous wound healing enhancement. J Invest Dermatol 2008;128:1565–75.

96. Cianfarani F, Tommasi R, Failla CM, et al. Granulocyte/macrophage colony-stimulating factor treatment of human chronic ulcers promotes angiogenesis associated with de novo vascular endothelial growth factor transcription in the ulcer bed. Br J Dermatol 2006;154:34–41.

97. Lu L, Saulis AS, Liu WR, et al. The temporal effects of anti-TGF-beta1, 2, and 3 monoclonal antibody on wound healing and hypertrophic scar formation. J Am Coll Surg 2005;201:391–7.

98. Geusens B, Sanders N, Prow T, et al. Cutaneous short-interfering RNA therapy. Expert Opin Drug Deliv 2009;6:1333–49.

99. Lu PY, Xie F, Woodle MC. In vivo application of RNA interference: from functional genomics to therapeutics. Adv Genet 2005;54:117–42.

Regenerative Materials That Facilitate Wound Healing

Gerit Mulder, DPM, MS, PhD, FRCST, MAPWCA[a],*,
Kelly Wallin, DPM[b], Mayer Tenenhaus, MD[c]

KEYWORDS

- Wound healing • Regenerative materials • Acellular materials • Allografts • Xenografts
- Living skin equivalents • Skin ulcers • Matrices

KEY POINTS

- The primary role of regenerative products is not to act as autologous skin graft, but to provide a means of dynamic interaction in the wound bed, thereby assisting and promoting tissue regeneration and wound closure.
- The clinician needs to differentiate between patients with normal and active cell responses versus those with impaired cellular activity, to assist with the choice of a living cell versus an acellular product.
- Not all acellular products function, integrate, or respond in the same manner, as a result of the variability of materials, structure, and components in each type of matrix.
- The variety and selection of regenerative materials, recently referred to as biomodulators, is so large that it has become necessary to classify them as either drugs, cellular products, or acellular products.

REGENERATIVE MATERIALS THAT FACILITATE WOUND HEALING

The treatment of problematic and chronic wounds has evolved in the last 3 decades, progressing from the introduction of the first simple occlusive dressings[1,2] to drugs and biologic materials. The addition of regenerative materials as well as biologic matrices has been a more recent addition to treatment modalities for wounds that do not respond to standard, conventional approaches for wound care. The rapid development and growth of cellular and acellular tissue replacements, matrices, and engineered products designed specifically for use in problematic wounds occurred after the introduction of living cell equivalents more than a decade ago.[3,4] Since then, numerous acellular materials have been introduced and studied for use in tissue repair.[5]

The variety and selection of regenerative materials, recently referred to as biomodulators, is currently so large that it has become necessary to classify them as either drugs, cellular products, or acellular products.

This article focuses on the use of true matrix replacements, including living cell and acellular wound materials. Applications of these types of products may extend beyond wound healing and are applicable to ulcers, tendon repair, hernia repair, tissue augmentation and other internal uses. This article discusses only the uses in wound healing in acute, chronic, and problematic wounds.

It is important to recognize that the primary role of regenerative products is not to act as autologous skin graft; they are designed to provide a means of dynamic interaction in the wound bed, thereby assisting and promoting tissue regeneration and

[a] Division of Trauma, Department of Surgery, Wound Treatment and Research Center, University of California San Diego, 200 West Arbor Drive #8896, San Diego, CA 92103-8896, USA; [b] Mercy Medical Center, San Diego, 4077 Fifth Avenue, San Diego, CA 92103, USA; [c] Department of Surgery, Division of Plastic Surgery, University of California at San Diego Medical Center, Hillcrest 200 West Arbor Drive, San Diego, CA 92103, USA
* Corresponding author.
E-mail address: gmulder01@aol.com

Clin Plastic Surg 39 (2012) 249–267
doi:10.1016/j.cps.2012.05.006
0094-1298/12/$ – see front matter Published by Elsevier Inc.

wound closure. The term that best describes this process, biomodulation, was first used during an International Consensus on Acellular Matrices for the Treatment of Wounds.[6]

The Extracellular Matrix

The extracellular matrix (ECM) is a key component of the tissue repair process. Its composition includes:

- Fibronectin
- Elastin
- Collagen
- Proteoglycans
- Hyaluronic acid.

The ECM is best compared with the framework or skeletal structure of a building in which all other components are added to the basic foundation and framework. Growth factors, fibroblasts, and other cellular components depend on the ECM for ongoing activity and tissue regeneration. The absence of an adequate ECM may significantly impair the natural sequence of tissue repair. The need for the presence of a matrix and regeneration in a wound bed has led to the development of regenerative products with a three-dimensional matrix (with or without a living cell component) that provide the framework for the repair process.

Most of the currently available materials are:

- Animal-derived or human-derived processed tissue
- Collagen-based or hyaluronic-based dressings
- Synthetic products
- Chemical constructs.

Living cells can also be used in conjunction with synthetic or collagen-based constructs. Because of the source of materials, many of these products are classified as biologic by the US Food and Drug Administration (FDA) (animal, human, or plant derived[7]).

Regardless of the manufacturing process, the tissue replacements and regenerative matrices are not antimicrobial agents. When placed in tissue defects that are not sterile or surgical uncontaminated wounds, bacterial growth becomes a barrier to effectiveness and outcomes. Aggressive debridement is needed to remove all nonviable and contaminated tissue. High levels of bacterial burden are known to impair the repair process, increase protease activity, and lead to further tissue breakdown.[8,9] Most regenerative materials are protein based, therefore they are sensitive to protease levels, which may contribute to rapid degradation. Bacteria may also proliferate in a matrix and contribute to wound infection and

---

> **Creating an optimal environment for regenerative products: key points**
>
> 1. Remove all nonviable tissue
> 2. Create a clean, bacteria-free environment
> 3. Control the level of inflammation
> 4. Protect product from external contamination
> 5. Consider the concomitant use of antimicrobial agents

---

further increase of matrix metalloproteinases (MMPs). Before application of any the products discussed in this article, bacterial presence must be significantly reduced or eliminated. The optimal environment for application of a wound matrix or regenerative product is the surgical setting, in which excisional and full-thickness debridement may be performed without difficulty. After application, protection from outside contamination, antibiotic use, and topical antimicrobials should always be considered to prevent new colonization or proliferation.

When choosing to use any newer technology, which inevitably comes with a significantly higher cost, clinicians should determine whether there are sufficient data to support the use of the product instead of more conventional modalities, and whether less expensive conventional treatments may provide similar results and time to wound closure.

LIVING CELL PRODUCTS

Cellular-derived wound healing products contain living cells such as fibroblasts, keratinocytes, or stem cells that are commonly embedded within a collagen or polyglactin matrix. Living cell products are designed to simulate the functional and biologic properties of human skin by:

- Providing a mechanical barrier to infection
- Encouraging extracellular matrix formation
- Stimulating keratinocyte growth and differentiation.

Living cell products are indicated for burn wounds, epidermolysis bullosa (EB), and most chronic wounds including diabetic, venous, and pressure wounds.

Only a few live-cell products are approved for clinical use (**Table 1**). It is important for the clinician to understand the indications for each product and carefully evaluate any potential barriers to healing, such as infection, comorbidities, or patient noncompliance, to provide the best possible clinical

Table 1
Live-cell wound products available in the United States/Europe

Product	Company	Description	Live Cells	Uses
Apligraf	Organogenesis, Inc, Canton, MA	Bilayered epidermal and dermal equivalent	Neonatal keratinocytes	Chronic wounds: venous, diabetic
Dermagraft	Advanced Biohealing, Inc, La Jolla, CA	Single-layered dermal equivalent	Neonatal fibroblasts	Chronic diabetic wounds
Epicel	Genzyme Tissue Repair Corp, Cambridge, MA	Cultured autologous keratinocytes	Autogenous keratinocytes	Burn wounds >30% TBSA
Laserskin	Fidia Advanced Biopolymers, Abano Terme, Italy	Cultured autologous keratinocytes	Autogenous keratinocytes	Burn wounds >30% TBSA

Abbreviation: TBSA: total body surface area.

outcome. Wounds of different cause, depth, age, and surface area must be treated differently and have dissimilar clinical prognoses. The use of adjunctive therapies such as compression, off-loading, and antibiotics should always be considered, if appropriate, to maximize healing success. Because living cell products are sensitive to bacteria and proteases, aggressive debridement is important, but only in the presence of adequate blood flow and the absence of any contraindication to sharp surgical debridement.

Wound Healing in Chronic Wounds

Normal wound healing requires a timely cellular response to injury by activation of keratinocytes, fibroblasts, endothelial cells, macrophages, and platelets, with resultant intercellular signaling through the coordinated release of growth factors and cytokines.[10] Most chronic wounds are 1 of 3 categories:

1. Pressure sores
2. Diabetic ulcers
3. Venous ulcers.

Prolonged chronic wounds have been shown to be deficient in growth factors (epidermal growth factor receptor, keratinocyte growth factor, platelet derived growth factor [PDGF] and insulinlike growth factor [IGF]) and display[11]:

- Decreased keratinocyte and fibroblast migration
- Increased reactive oxygen species
- Increased tissue proteases
- Microbial contamination.

Normal dermal fibroblasts synthesize and deposit critical extracellular components as well as secreting key growth factors important for intercellular signaling and repair. Fibroblasts from chronic wounds show pathologic changes in morphology, growth, and gene expression and have decreased or nonexistent replicative and functional ability.[12] Keratinocytes are similarly dysfunctional, losing the ability to migrate from the wound edges and re-epithelialize the wound surface.[13] These key cells eventually become senescent and lose the capacity to react to growth factors that would normally stimulate a healing response.[14]

Wound Healing in Diabetes

Wound healing in the diabetic patient is particularly challenging, because diabetic ulcers are slow to heal and prone to more serious complications such as osteomyelitis and amputation.[15–17] There are more than 100 known physiologic factors that contribute to wound healing deficiencies in the diabetic patient, including[18–20]:

- Derangement of cellular systems responsible for growth factor function
- Angiogenic response
- Macrophage function
- Collagen formation
- Epidermal barrier function
- Granulation tissue formation.

Regardless of the specific cause, it is vital to restore the continuity and integrity of the damaged skin in a timely fashion to minimize further morbidity and prevent complication. Regenerative live-cell products are designed to mimic the inherent cellular properties of the skin and provide temporary supplementation of critical functions lost by the chronic wound, such as keratinocyte and fibroblast proliferation and differentiation, extracellular matrix synthesis, and eventual reepithelialization.

The clinician needs to differentiate between patients with normal and active cell responses versus those with impaired cellular activity, to assist with the choice of a living cell versus an acellular product.

Apligraf

Apligraf (Organogenesis, Inc, Canton, MA, USA) is a bilayered skin equivalent designed to replicate the normal skin's epidermis and dermis. The epidermal equivalent layer consists of a neonatal keratinocyte layer that is exposed to oxygen during the manufacturing process, giving rise to a stratified monolayer similar to the stratum corneum. The dermal equivalent layer contains neonatal fibroblasts impregnated on an extracellular collagen matrix composed of both bovine and human type I collagen. It is void of antigenic cells such as Langerhans cells, melanocytes, lymphocytes, macrophages, hair follicles, blood vessels, or sweat glands. Although the mechanism of action is not fully understood, it is thought that Apligraf creates a microenvironment that provides a physical and biologic barrier against wound infection and also produces a variety of MMPs, cytokines, and growth factors responsible for keratinocyte migration and extracellular matrix formation.[21,22]

Use and Application of Apligraf

Apligraf is approved by the FDA for chronic venous ulcers of greater than 1 month's duration and for diabetic ulcers of more than 3 weeks' duration.

- It is supplied as a circular disk with a diameter of 7.5 cm and is 0.75 mm thick.
- It has a shelf life of 10 days and must be stored at 20 to 23°C until used.
- Apligraf may be applied every 4 to 6 weeks depending on the wound type, location, and clinician preference.
- As with most graft applications, wound bed preparation is critical and must involve proper debridement and control of edema and infection.
- Apligraf can be meshed or slit to facilitate drainage and is laid flat directly over the wound bed with the dermal side (glossy side) down.
- The graft should overlap the wound margin by 2 to 3 mm and care should be taken to smooth any wrinkles or air pockets. The graft is secured in place with staples or adhesive strips and protected with a soft primary dressing.
- Application of the product to the plantar diabetic foot requires special off-loading precautions to prevent disruption with ambulation.
- When applied to venous ulcers, compression is still required to address venous return. Compression needs to be applied carefully to prevent product disruption.

Apligraf Studies

Chronic venous leg ulcers

In 2000, Falanga[23] published a prospective, randomized study of 214 patients with chronic venous leg ulcers treated with Apligraf with compression therapy versus compression therapy alone. Those patients treated with Apligraf were 3 times more likely to heal wounds older than 1 year ($P = .008$) and 2 times more likely to attain complete wound healing by 24 weeks ($P = .002$).

Diabetic foot ulcers

Veves and colleagues[3] studied 208 patients in a multicenter, randomized, controlled trial in 2001 that compared Apligraf with moist gauze dressings for the treatment of diabetic foot ulcers. At 12 weeks, 56% of patients treated with Apligraf had complete wound healing versus 38% in the control group ($P = .004$). The Apligraf-treated patients also had a faster median wound closure time of 65 days versus 90 days ($P = .003$).

EB

Apligraf has also been used in the treatment of EB. Fivenson and colleagues published a small study of 9 patients with 96 sites of skin loss, of which, 90% to 100% healing was observed by 5 to 7 days, with clinically normal-appearing skin present by days 10 to 14. Falabella and colleagues[24] also reported success in treating 69 acute EB wounds with no adverse events related to the application of Apligraf.

Dermagraft Dermagraft (Advanced Biohealing, Inc, La Jolla, CA, USA) is a cryopreserved, single-layered, dermal substitute containing human-derived neonatal fibroblasts cultured on a bioresorbable polyglactin 910 scaffold. It stimulates the ingrowth of fibrovascular and epithelial tissue by depositing extracellular matrix components such as collagens, vitronectin, and glycosaminoglycans, and also secretes a variety of cytokines and growth factors including vascular endothelial growth factor (VEGF), PDGF, IGF-1, and granulocyte/macrophage colony-stimulating factor (GM-CSF). The fibroblasts continue to secrete growth factors and recruit host cells until fibrovascular ingrowth gradually replaces the donor cells and tissue. Dermagraft is void of antigenic cells and does not seem to stimulate rejection.

Use and Application

Dermagraft is primarily indicated and approved for the treatment of full-thickness diabetic foot ulcers of more than 6 weeks' duration that are not overlying bone, tendon, muscle, or joint capsule.

- Dermagraft is cryopreserved and must be stored at −70 to −80°C until ready for use
- It is supplied in a clear bag containing 1 piece approximately 5 cm × 7.5 cm
- The graft must be thawed by submerging in water at 34 to 37°C for approximately 2 minutes and can be held aside in saline for up to 30 minutes
- The graft is laid flat on the wound bed (either side of the graft may be placed down) and trimmed to the approximate circumference of the wound margins
- Care should be taken to smooth out any wrinkles or air pockets to maximize surface area contact
- The graft is secured in place with staples or adhesive strips and a soft primary dressing should be applied directly over the graft
- Control of edema or proper off-loading is accomplished with an appropriate secondary dressing
- The primary dressing should be left in place for a minimum of 72 hours
- Dermagraft can be applied weekly for a total of 8 applications over a 12-week period
- When applying Dermagraft to the plantar diabetic foot, off-loading and removal of all pressure from the wound site is imperative to prevent disruption of the material when ambulating.

Dermagraft Studies

Diabetic foot ulcers of more than 6 weeks' duration

Dermagraft was approved by the FDA in September 2001. The pivotal Dermagraft study was a multicenter, randomized, controlled study of 314 patients published by Marston and colleagues[4] that compared Dermagraft with conventional wound care methods over 12 weeks. Patients included in the final analysis had ulcers of greater than 6 weeks' duration. Twenty-eight percent of patients treated with Dermagraft achieved complete healing versus 14% in the control group ($P = .035$). Wounds were 1.6 to 1.7 times more likely to heal in the Dermagraft group and the median wound closure was 91% versus 78% in the control group ($P = .44$). The incidence of ulcer-related adverse events was also lower in the Dermagraft group (19%) compared with the control (32%; $P = .007$). Other non–FDA-approved uses included venous ulcers, fasciotomy wounds, buccal fat pad donor site healing, pediatric postsurgical abdominal wound healing, and vestibuloplasty.[25]

Cultured epidermal autograft A cultured epidermal autograft (CEA) is a single-layered epidermal substitute comprising the patient's own keratinocytes, which are cultured ex vivo, together with mouse fibroblasts to form a thin sheet of skin.[26] The total body surface area of a human (1.8 m²) can be produced in just 4 weeks, although minimum required preparation time for normal-sized wounds is 16 days. CEAs must be used in conjunction with a dermal substitute, which makes it fragile. It is currently approved for full-thickness burns of total body surface area greater than 30% and large congenital nevus excisions, although some success has been reported with treatment of leg ulcers.[27,28] Although CEAs have shown some limited success with burn wounds,[29] most of the literature concludes that it is generally unpredictable and inconsistent and should be used as an adjunct to conventional burn wound coverage with split-thickness autografts.[30] Various improvements to cultured epidermal autografts are currently being studied, including a hyaluronic acid membrane carrier and a spray-on application.[31,32]

The Future

Pilot studies are underway for the development of new live-cell regenerative wound care products. One such possibility is the use of multipotent adult stem cells, which have shown promise in

---

Using living cell products: key points

1. In the absence of contraindications and the presence of adequate blood flow for healing, debride the wound bed of all nonviable tissue
2. Ensure that the material is in full contact with the wound bed and apply a nonadhesive wound contact layer over the product before dressing
3. Securely attach the material to the wound margins
4. Address non–weight bearing, compression, and other related treatment factors
5. Avoid disruption of the dressing for up to 1 week if possible

accelerating wound repair and reconstituting the wound bed. Although considerable focus has been placed on bone marrow–derived mesenchymal stem cells, other types of stem cells are being studied, including those derived from hair follicles and adipose tissue.[33–38] Currently there are no FDA-approved products available, and randomized clinical trials are still needed.

ACELLULAR MATRICES

Acellular matrices are approved for use in most chronic wounds including diabetic, venous, and pressure ulcers; surgically dehisced wounds; and acute and chronic wounds. They may be classified as:

1. Allografts: human tissue
2. Xenografts: animal derived
3. Chemical constructs: may contain animal-derived collagen in additional to chemical components.

The large number and variety of acellular products is listed in **Table 2**. The increased interest in, and use of, regenerative materials has resulted in products being introduced into the market on a regular basis. **Table 2** reflects only those products that were available at the time this writing was completed.

Reviewing the list of acellular materials provides an insight into the variability of materials, structure, and components featured in each type of matrix. It is important for the clinician to understand that not all products function, integrate, or respond in the same manner.

- Ideally, a material is needed that is most similar to natural or native dermal matrices, thereby allowing cells to integrate and divide as they would in a natural host
- The function of the matrix is also determined by its physical placement and location; for example, an acellular matrix is placed in a large defect to allow for cell migration into the material while further acting as a chemoattractant
- The final anticipated result is rapid granulation leading to wound closure
- The quality of regenerated host tissue with its resulting tensile strength, turgor, and degree of scarring is also determined by the speed and manner in which wound repair occurred.

In summary, these materials may not necessarily function as expected, although it is anticipated that they may:

- Promote angiogenesis
- Provide a framework for cell migration and integration
- Act as chemoattractants
- Bind proteases
- Contain growth factors to promote healing
- Have receptors to bind fibroblasts.

To promote appropriate product selection, clinicians must have a basic understanding of the differences between products and what to select for the type of wound they are treating. Following are primary considerations in using regenerative matrices.

Sterilization

Regenerative matrices are either clean processed or fully sterile. This option has also been described as aseptically cleaned versus terminally sterilized. Aseptic cleansing does not guarantee the removal of all viral contamination and does carry a risk of hepatitis or human immunodeficiency virus transmission. Cadaver-derived tissue may be either aseptically cleaned or terminally sterilized depending on the manufacturer. The disadvantage of the more common terminal sterilization techniques is that they may damage and change the collagen structure of the product, rendering it more susceptible to rapid degradation.[39] High levels of MMPs in chronic wounds associated with inflammation, high levels of bacterial burden, and repetitive trauma, more easily degrade a product with denatured collagen or without heavy cross-linkage.

Structure

Matrices may be of human, animal, or synthetic origin. Careful review of the product literature prevents selection of a product that may be problematic for wound repair.

- Human tissue is closed to the natural matrix but may not be terminally sterilized or structurally strong.
- Cross-linkage may be weak and rapid degradation is likely to occur in the chronic wound environment.
- Transmission of virus, as previously mentioned, is a serious consideration.
- Animal products, particular certain porcine materials, may contain remaining host DNA fragments, which are known to induce a higher host inflammatory response as well as increased presence of giant cells.[9,40,41] The increased inflammatory reaction is of particular relevance if the material is being considered as an implant versus a topical biologically active cover.

Table 2
Acellular wound matrix products available in the United States/Europe

Xenograft Collagen Grafts

Manufacturer	Product	Source	Indicated For — Acute Wounds	Indicated For — Chronic Wounds	Shelf Life[a]/Storage	Cross-Linking	Sterilization Process
Acell Inc/Medline	MatriStem Wound Care Matrix	Porcine urinary bladder matrix	+	+	2 y at room temperature	None	Electron beam irradiation
AM Scientifics/Brennen Medical	EZ-DERM	Porcine dermis	+	+	Room temperature	Aldehyde	Sterile (method undocumented)
Cook Medical	Biodesign (Surgisis) Hernia Graft	Porcine small intestine submucosa	+	−	18 mo room temperature	None	Ethylene oxide
Covidien	Permacol	Porcine dermis	+	−	Room temperature	HDMI	γ Irradiation
Davol Inc/Bard	CollaMenc[a] Implant	Porcine dermis	+	−	Room temperature	EDC	Ethylene oxide
Davol Inc/Bard	XenMatrix Surgical Graft	Porcine dermis	+	−	Room temperature	None	Electron beam irradiation
Dr Suwelack Skin & Health Care AG/Eurosurgical	MATRIDERM	Bovine dermis	+	+	5 y Room temperature	None	γ Irradiation
Dr Suwelack Skin & Health Care AG/Medline	Puracol Plus Microscaffold Collagen (Puracol Plus Ag)	Bovine collagen (plus antimicrobial Ag)	+	+	3 y Room temperature	None	Supplied sterile (method undocumented)
Euroresearch	BIOPAD Collagen Wound Dressing Note: Biospray also available for minor burns and superficial wounds	Equine flexor tendon	+	+	Store in a dry place away from heat sources	None	γ Irradiation
Healthpoint Ltd/Cook Biotech, Inc	OASIS Wound Matrix	Porcine small intestine submucosa	+	+	2 y room temperature	None	Ethylene oxide
Integra LifeSciences	INTEGRA Matrix Wound Dressing	Bovine tendon collagen and glycosaminoglycan	+	+	2 y room temperature	Glutaraldehyde	Ethylene oxide

(continued on next page)

Table 2
(continued)

Manufacturer	Product	Source	Indicated For		Shelf Life[a]/Storage	Cross-Linking	Sterilization Process
			Acute Wounds	Chronic Wounds			
LifeCell	Strattice Reconstructive Tissue Matrix	Porcine dermis	+	−	Room temperature	None	Electron beam irradiation
Mesynthes	Endoform Dermal Template	Propria-submucosa layers of bovine forestomach	+	+	Room temperature	None	Ethylene oxide
Synovis Orthopedic and Woundcare, Inc	Unite Biomatrix Collagen Wound Dressing	Equine pericardium	+	+	3 y room temperature	EDC	EDC
Synovis Orthopedic and Woundcare, Inc	Veritas Collagen Matrix	Bovine pericardium	+	−	Controlled room temperature	None	Sodium hydroxide
TEI Biosciences	PriMatrix Dermal Repair Scaffold	Fetal bovine dermis	+	+	3 y room temperature	None	Ethylene oxide
TEI Biosciences	SurgiMend/ SurgiMend Inguinal Hernia Repair Matrix	Fetal bovine dermis	+	−	3 y room temperature	None	Ethylene oxide
Allografts							
ADI Medical/HANS Biomed	SureDerm Acellular Dermal Graft	Human dermis	+	−	2 y refrigeration necessary	None	Supplied sterile
Davol Inc/Bard	AlloMax Surgical Graft	Human dermis	+	−	No refrigeration required	None	Tutoplast process and low-dose γ Irradiation
LifeCell	AlloDerm Regenerative Tissue Matrix Also available as a micronized version (Cymetra)	Human dermis	+	−	2 y freeze dried, refrigerate on receipt	None	Aseptically processed
Mentor	NeoForm	Human dermis	+	−	5 y room temperature	None	Tutoplast process and low-dose γ Irradiation

Musculoskeletal Transplant Foundation/ Ethicon	FlexHD Acellular Hydrated Dermis	Human dermis	+	−	Ready to use, room temperature	None	Aseptically processed (passes the US Pharmacopeia Standard 71 for sterility)
Musculoskeletal Transplant Foundation/ Synthes CMF	DermaMatrix Acellular Dermis	Human dermis	+	−	3 y freeze dried Room temperature	None	Aseptically processed (passes the US Pharmacopeia Standard 71 for sterility)
Wright Medical Technology, Inc	GRAFTJACKET Regenerative Tissue Matrix Ulcer Repair Also available as a micronized version (GRAFTJACKET Xpress Flowable Soft-Tissue Scaffold)	Human dermis	+	+	2 y freeze dried, refrigerate on receipt	None	Aseptically processed
Synthetic Acellular Dermal Replacements							
Integra LifeSciences	INTEGRA Bilayer Matrix Wound Dressing	Bilayered: bovine tendon collagen and glycosaminoglycan with a polysiloxane (silicone) membrane	+	+	2 y room temperature	Aqueous glutaraldehyde	Irradiation
Integra LifeSciences	INTEGRA Dermal Regeneration Template	Bilayered: bovine tendon collagen and glycosaminoglycan with a polysiloxane (silicone) membrane	+	−	2 y, store flat and refrigerate	Glutaraldehyde	γ Irradiation

All information has been checked against manufacturers' Web sites. Please refer to individual product literature for use.

a Shelf life is cited when known.

The rate of degradation in a chronic wound, although influenced by the aforementioned factors, is further affected by the degree and type of cross-linkage. Not all products are cross-linked in a similar fashion. The manufacturing process, sterilization, and the physical characteristics of the material used determine the resulting cross-linkage of a product. Non–cross-linked materials are likely to be rapidly absorbed, whereas heavily cross-linked materials remain more resistant to breakdown. Even cross-linked materials vary in whether the bonds are rigid or flexible. Cell migration is facilitated by the absence of cross-linking or flexible links versus rigid cross-linking. Chemical or synthetic products are sterile, non–cross-linked, and rapidly resorbed.[42,43]

The choice of which material to use is based on the wound cause, wound characteristics, and desired outcome. A clean full-thickness wound not requiring extensive debridement that is to undergo a split-thickness or other graft may benefit from a chemical construct or acellular graft, which allows rapid cell migration. The goal with a wound in which autologous grafting is the end point is rapid cell integration and resulting granulation, thereby decreasing the time before a wound bed is ready for a graft. In such cases, expediting granulation and decreasing time to a graft-ready wound bed is important in decreasing the time to surgery intended to fully close a wound, particularly in high-risk and immunocompromised patients. Heavy or rigid cross-linked materials are not desirable in this scenario. Granulation seems to be further expedited through the use of negative-pressure wound therapy.[44]

The selection of a more cross-linked product is appropriate in wounds in which inflammation is high, as is the case in patients with vasculitis and other autoimmune diseases.

An additional and important consideration before application is the source of the product (**Box 1**). Acellular materials may be human or animal derived (bovine, porcine, equine). Allergies to animal products, as well as cultural issues, must be considered.

Standard Care Versus Advanced Technologies: Considerations for Use

Advanced technologies, including regenerative materials, are associated with a higher financial burden compared with conventional dressings and approaches to wound care. Regenerative tissues and matrices may sound appealing, but require scientific and clinical evidence to justify their use in the current financially burdened medical environment.

Individuals with wounds that are progressing to closure, without factors impairing the normal repair process and with acute wounds, may be expected to respond well to conventional dressings and treatments. Most patients are still best treated with less expensive and basic dressings and wound care. Following are considerations for use of regenerative materials.

Inability to generate a wound matrix

Regenerative materials and wound matrices are excellent options in patients unable to effectively or rapidly generate a wound matrix. The matrix is needed as a scaffold to support:

- Cell ingrowths
- Cell differentiation
- Binding of cells to receptors
- Chemoattraction of cells and other growth factors
- Angiogenesis
- Wound bed granulation.

Regenerative materials may support some or all of these properties.

Wound repair, not disease treatment

Underlying disease and wound cause must be addressed if successful outcomes are to be expected. Regenerative tissues are designed to address the

---

Box 1
Considerations for selecting the appropriate product

1. Acellular products are either clean processed or sterilized. A sterilized product is always preferable.

2. The degree of cross-linkage affects the ability of cells to migrate into the product as well as the ability of proteases to degrade the product.

3. Acellular products may be bovine, porcine, equine, or human in origin. Take into consideration allergies and cultural beliefs.

4. High protease levels affect the degradation of a product. Determine the expected degree of inflammation in the wound bed.

5. Products may be placed in a wound as a matrix or over a wound with negative-pressure wound therapy, so choose a product that allows rapid cell integration and fenestration for passage of exudate.

wound defect and repair process, not the disease state. Before application of any regenerative materials, the physician must address:

- Diabetes control
- Adequate vascular supply
- Control of infection
- Bacterial burden
- Medical attention to the patient's primary disease states.

Additional factors to consider before applying a regenerative material include:

- Patient eligibility
- Vascular status
- Ability to undergo aggressive debridement
- Healing potential
- Ability to maintain sterility at wound site
- Wound size
- Wound drainage
- Periwound edema
- Level of patient activity and ambulation
- Ability to control the patient's disease states.

Securing the material
A final consideration is the ability to secure the product, whether with sutures, staples, or adhesive strips. Products that are not in full contact with the wound bed allow disruption of the material, accumulation of exudate, and an environment promoting bacterial growth.

What are the advantages of regenerative materials? These include creating an environment conducive to wound closure, supplying a matrix in a defect where one is not present, expediting granulation, facilitating cell migration into a wound bed, increasing angiogenesis, chemoattractant properties, and a reduced time to wound closure.[6,45–47]

What are the disadvantages of regenerative materials? These include high short-term costs (long-term cost of care may be reduced and considered an advantage), high potential for product contamination and infection, need for aggressive wound bed preparation, high failure rate with inappropriate handling, and need for a higher level of education and training of the clinician. Use of antimicrobial agents or secondary dressings should be considered to reduce risk of contamination progressing to a true clinical infection.

Is the product used as a true matrix/scaffold or a biologic cover? Consider whether the chosen product is being used as a true matrix or scaffold, which is to remain in the wound until full closure, or whether it is to act as a biologic cover. Know what to expect when applying the product.

- A deep defect may require a material that allows rapid cell integration, rapid product degradation, and coverage with secondary dressings.
- A wound that is not closing because of reduced cell activity or presence of high levels of MMPs may benefit from a regenerative tissue being used as a biologic modulating cover to alter the wound environment to one that is favorable rather than destructive.
- The chronic wound that does not progress to closure may have potential from a cellular level but does not have potential from an environmental perspective. Controlling lifestyle, activities, and compliance is especially challenging in the patient with a chronic wound. Off-loading may be particularly difficult with the ambulatory diabetic patient.

Pairing product with a wound
Variability among wounds, even those of a similar cause, is difficult because all wounds vary in depth, exudate, bacterial burden, location, and presentation. Only general recommendations may be made concerning the appropriate choice of product. General rules provide guidelines; however, individual variation must be considered.

- Wounds associated with high levels of inflammation, including vasculitic and inflammatory ulcers, respond better to products that are highly cross-linked, because this reduces the rate of degradation. The negative feature of rigid cross-linking is the barrier created to cell migration; however, a flexible cross-linkage allows cells to migrate into the matrix with less difficulty. See cases 1 and 2.
- If rapid granulation is desired, as with wounds being prepared for grafting, a chemical construct without cross-linkage is more appropriate because cells will migrate without difficulty, the product will degrade rapidly,

---

Patient considerations when using regenerative products: key points

1. Underlying disease process must be controlled
2. Patient requires adequate vascular flow for healing
3. Wound must be able to undergo aggressive debridement
4. Wound must be free of infection
5. Patient's wound must come into full contact with the surface of the product to reduce risk of fluid accumulation and infection

---

Case 1: Xenograft for lesions unresponsive to conservative care and surgery

Figs. 1–3 show a patient with multiple diseases associated with inflammation, including antiphospholipid syndrome and Raynaud phenomenon as well as vasculitis, who had a history of painful lesions unresponsive to all forms of conservative care as well as surgical intervention with skin grafts.

- A flexible cross-linked equine pericardium material was placed over the wound following hydrosurgical debridement in the operating room.
- The xenograft was attached with adhesive strips to avoid further irritation incurred by removal of staples. The secondary dressings were changed once a week.
- Within 2 weeks, the outer portion of the xenograft desiccated and presented as an eschar. In such cases, the product seems to biomodulate underlying cellular activity while binding destructive proteases. Once the xenograft presented as an eschar, the patient was allowed to shower and dry the material and cover it with gauze.
- The patient had multiple bilateral extremity wounds that all headed within 12 weeks after having been present for 5 years.
- She remains pain free and without lesions 2 years after the procedure.

The black discoloration over the material is the result of a secondary nanocrystalline silver dressing used to prevent external contamination.

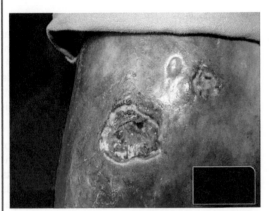

Fig. 1. Patient with vasculitis, antiphospholipid syndrome, and Raynaud phenomenon with multiple leg wounds present for greater than 5 years, unresponsive to previous conservative and surgical interventions.

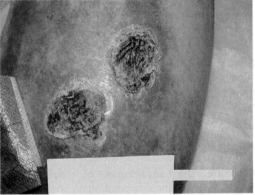

Fig. 2. Patient 5 weeks after application of xenograft. Xenograft desiccated and attached to wound bed. As xenograft separates, margins may be trimmed. Dark discoloration is from silver dressing that had been placed over the wound.

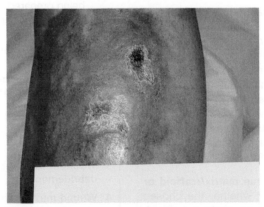

Fig. 3. Patient approximately 10 weeks after surgery when remaining xenografts have fallen off the wound, with underlying tissue completely healed.

Case 2: Xenograft for full-thickness plantar wound

In **Figs. 4–6**, a young woman who underwent a motor vehicle accident with subsequent reconstruction of her foot presented with a large full-thickness wound in the plantar area. This area of the body is not easily addressed with grafts. Daily or frequent dressing changes are extremely painful. Use of a xenograft (in this case, a fenestrated, flexible, cross-linked, sterile, equine xenograft) allowed a single application surgically, followed by weekly changes of the outer antimicrobial nanocrystalline silver dressing, and non–weight bearing.

Because the patient was non–weight bearing and on crutches, the material was attached with adhesive strips, although staples could have been used. The patient was ambulatory at postoperative week 3, with complete healing and minimal scarring at week 5, when only a small wound remained, closing in 1 more week with traditional dressings. The patient had minimal to no pain during the course of healing.

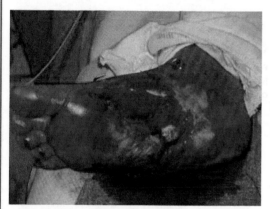

Fig. 4. Trauma on the plantar foot resulting in a large plantar defect that could not easily be closed during surgery with skin grafting or flap.

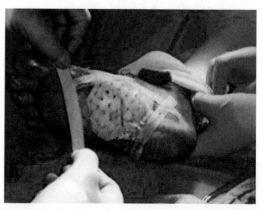

Fig. 5. Application of a fenestrated equine pericardium xenograft attached with adhesive strips used as the patient is non–weight bearing and staple removal could be painful in this area. The wound is subsequently covered with a nonadherent silver-impregnated petrolatum wound contact dressing, bolstered gauze, and gauze wrap. Only the outer gauze is changed weekly.

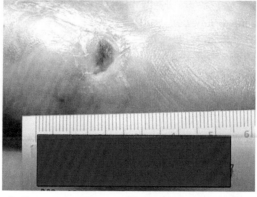

Fig. 6. Five weeks after application, the remaining xenograft detaches revealing a small wound, approximately 0.4 × 0.6 cm, that is effectively treated with a topical dressing. The patient is now ambulatory in a walking boot, with minimal pain, and able to shower without difficulty. There is minimal periwound scarring evident.

Case 3: Open ankle fracture using split-thickness skin graft over Integra graft

Figs. 7–11.

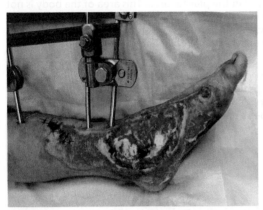

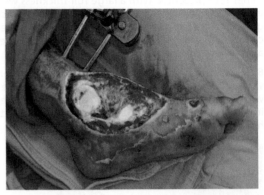

Fig. 7. Open ankle fracture in a 10-year-old girl. (Case and figures *courtesy of* Mark Granick, MD.)

Fig. 8. Wound debrided with a VERSAJET (Smith and Nephew, Largo, FL, USA). (Case and figures *courtesy of* Mark Granick, MD.)

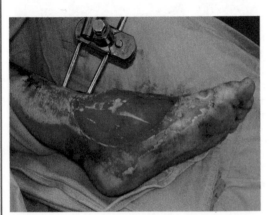

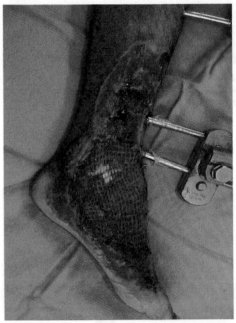

Fig. 9. Integra (Integra Life Sciences, Nutley, NJ, USA) placed over the wound. (Case and figures *courtesy of* Mark Granick, MD.)

Fig. 10. Meshed split-thickness skin graft placed over the mature Integra graft. (Case and figures *courtesy of* Mark Granick, MD.)

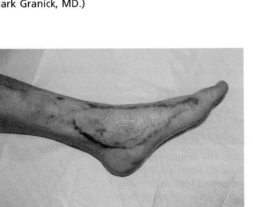

Fig. 11. The healed wound 2 years after surgery. (Case and figures *courtesy of* Mark Granick, MD.)

and a graft may be placed over the resulting healthy wound bed.

- In deep defects, particularly if negative pressure is used, a product with less cross-linkage is preferred. A product should be chosen that can be easily meshed to allow exudate to escape from the wound and not accumulate under the product.
- Materials that require weekly application because of associated rapid degradation are more suited for the outpatient setting, although a surgeon may choose to use these on more superficial exposed areas that are not closed by primary intention in the operating room.
- Wounds that are secondary to trauma, but present with a clean base, may be debrided and covered with a xenograft, which is left intact until complete healing occurs.

See case 3 for split-thickness skin graft over Integra graft in an open ankle wound.

Promising clinical results have been reported with synthetic tissue-engineered acellular matrix products such as MATRIDERM (Medskin Solutions, Germany). MATRIDERM is a three-dimensional, porous scaffold comprising both collagen and elastin, which serves as a framework by which autologous cells can migrate and colonize. MATRIDERM is a dermal substitute and is used in conjunction with a split-thickness skin graft for full-thickness wounds secondary to burns and trauma. See case 4.

Case 4: MATRIDERM and unmeshed split-thickness skin graft for a degloving injury

Figs. 12–15 show the case of a 71-year-old woman who sustained a degloving injury to the left lower extremity (see **Fig. 12**) with significant soft tissue loss and exposure of tendon and periosteum following operative debridement (see **Fig. 13**). Coverage was obtained using MATRIDERM and an unmeshed split-thickness skin graft with excellent take following 1 week of negative-pressure wound therapy (see **Fig. 14**). Two years after the injury, the patient was able to wear normal shoes and clinical gait analysis showed an excellent functional outcome (see **Fig. 15**).

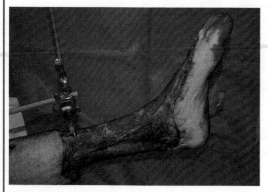

Fig. 12. Degloving injury.

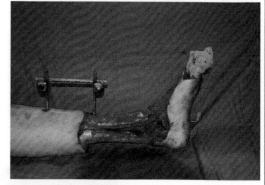

Fig. 13. After debridement.

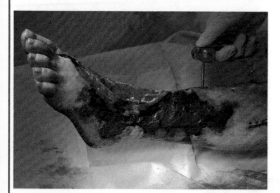

Fig. 14. Coverage with MATRIDERM and unmeshed split-thickness skin graft.

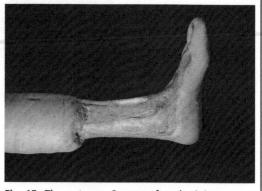

Fig. 15. The outcome 2 years after the injury.

Case 5: Split-thickness skin graft - Integra

Figs. 16–20.

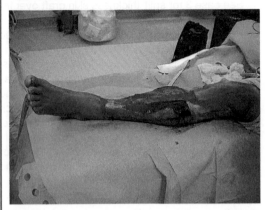

Fig. 16. Deep lower extremity burn following debridement. Tibia is exposed.

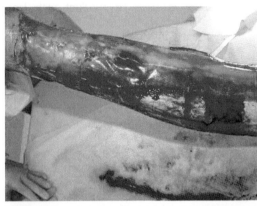

Fig. 17. Bilayer Integra placed over tibia (Integra Life Sciences, Nutley, NJ, USA).

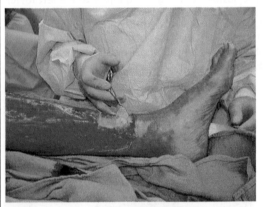

Fig. 18. The silicone layer is peeled off of the integrated graft.

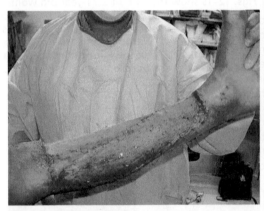

Fig. 19. Split thickness skin graft is applied to the wound.

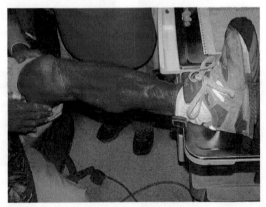

Fig. 20. The healed wound.

A few important recommendations for acellular matrices include:

- Debridement of all nonviable tissue
- Aggressive cleansing to remove bacterial burden
- Use of postoperative antibiotics for 10 days based on preoperative or intraoperative cultures (in the presence of bone infection, the product should not be applied)
- Coverage with a secondary antimicrobial dressing followed by bolstered gauze and wraps
- Pressure reduction or relief at the surgical site
- Minimal disruption of the dressings for 1-week periods.

Manufacturers cannot recommend use of antibiotics; however, the clinician may consider placing the allografts and certain xenografts in an antibiotic solution (based on suspected organisms) during the intraoperative procedure, for up to 20 minutes before application. Although there is no evidence to support this practice, any bacteria introduced on the wound surface or product is reasonably addressed by this treatment. However, bacteria remaining deep in the tissue may still contribute to infection. When graft materials become malodorous, overly moist, or separated, they need to be removed, because these are indicators of bacterial overgrowth.

Additional applications

This article focuses on the use of acellular matrices that assist with tissue generation for use in open wounds of all causes. The same materials may be used for tendon repair and other orthopedic use,[48] as well as for tissue augmentation. The reader is referred to the medical literature for information on use beyond wound repair. Growth factors may also be considered regenerative products. Becaplerim is an FDA-approved growth factor for the treatment of diabetic foot ulcers.[33] Although growth factors are considered regenerative, they are classified as drugs and not devices or biologic agents, therefore a discussion on their use has not been included. Stem cells are also considered regenerative and are being explored for use in chronic wounds.[34–38] Stem cells are considered a new area of clinical research and materials that may, in the future, be an additional form of treatment of problematic wounds.

SUMMARY

Regenerative materials, which include but are not limited to growth factors, cell products, collagen-based dressings, chemical constructs and acellular allografts, and xenografts are all designed to assist with the repair process when it is not occurring in an orderly and expected manner. This article focuses on the use of the acellular materials. Use of all the products discussed may be considered when the wound repair process is delayed, inhibited, or not progressing. Regenerative materials may be a primary choice when used in the surgical patient in whom postoperative complications may be expected if the wound is not covered with an interactive dressing. Careful patient selection, aggressive wound bed preparation, and close follow-up is recommended to ensure optimal results. The clinician or surgeon selecting these products needs a good understanding of differences between products, indications for use, and appropriate application techniques. When used as directed and when recommended, regenerative products may assist with expediting closure of recalcitrant wounds.

REFERENCES

1. Mulder GD, Albert SF, Grimwood RE. Clinical evaluation of a new occlusive hydrocolloid dressing. Cutis 1985;35(4):396–400.
2. Friedman SF, Su DW. Management of leg ulcers with hydrocolloid occlusive dressing. Arch Dermatol 1984;120(10):1329–36.
3. Veves A, Falanga V, Armstrong DG, et al. Graftskin, a human skin equivalent, is effective in the management of noninfected neuropathic diabetic foot ulcers: a prospective randomized multicenter clinical trial. Diabetes Care 2001;24(2):290–5.
4. Marston WA, Hanft J, Norwood P, et al, Dermagraft Diabetic Foot Ulcer Study Group. The efficacy and safety of Dermagraft in improving the healing of chronic diabetic foot ulcers: results of a prospective randomized trial. Diabetes Care 2003;26(6):1701–5.
5. Shevchenko RV, James SLL, Manes SE. A review of tissue-engineered skin bioconstructs available for skin reconstruction. J R Soc Interface 2010;7(48):229–58.
6. International consensus. Acellular matrices for the treatment of wounds. An expert working group review. London: Wounds International; 2010.
7. Section 201(h) of the Federal Food, Drug and Cosmetic Act (21 U.S.C. 321(h)).
8. Steed DC, Attinger C, Colaizzi T, et al. Guidelines for the treatment of diabetic ulcers. Wound Repair Regen 2006;14:680–92.
9. Browne AC, Vearncombe M, Sibbald GR. High bacterial load in asymptomatic diabetic patients with neuropathic ulcers retards wound healing of the application of Dermagraft. Ostomy Wound Manage 2001;47(10):44–9.

10. Singer AJ, Clark RA. Cutaneous wound healing. N Engl J Med 1999;341(10):738–46.

11. Mustoe T. Understanding chronic wounds: a unifying hypothesis on their pathogenesis and implications for therapy. Am J Surg 2004;187(5A):65S–70S.

12. Telgenhoff D, Shroot B. Cellular senescence mechanisms in chronic wound healing. Cell Death Differ 2005;12(7):695–8.

13. Bernard D, Gosselin K, Monte D, et al. Involvement of Rel/nuclear factor-kappaB transcription factors in keratinocyte senescence. Cancer Res 2004;64(2): 472–81.

14. Mulder GD, Vande Berg JS. Cellular senescence and matrix metalloproteinase activity in chronic wounds. Relevance to debridement and new technologies. J Am Podiatr Med Assoc 2002;92(1):34–7.

15. Brem H, Sheehan P, Boulton AJ. Protocol for treatment of diabetic foot ulcers [review]. Am J Surg 2004;187(5A):1S–10S.

16. Moss SE, Kelein R, Klein BE. The 14-year incidence of lower extremity amputations in a diabetic population: the Wisconsin Epidemiologic Study of Diabetic Retinopathy. Diabetes Care 1999;22: 951–9.

17. Frykberg RG, Armstrong DG, Giurini J, et al. Diabetic foot disorders: a clinical practice guideline. American College of Foot and Ankle Surgeons. J Foot Ankle Surg 2000;39:S1–60.

18. Galkowska H, Wojewodzka U, Olszewski WL. Chemokines, cytokines, and growth factors in keratinocytes and dermal endothelial cells in the margin of chronic diabetic foot ulcers. Wound Repair Regen 2006;14(5):558–65.

19. Falanga V. Wound healing and its impairment in the diabetic foot. Lancet 2005;366(9498):1736–43.

20. Brem H, Tomic-Canic M. Cellular and molecular basis of wound healing in diabetes. J Clin Invest 2007;117(5):1219–22.

21. Zaulyanov L, Kirsner RS. A review of a bi-layered living cell treatment (Apligraf) in the treatment of venous leg ulcers and diabetic foot ulcers. Clin Interv Aging 2007;2(1):93–8.

22. Ehrenreich M, Ruszczak Z. Update on tissue-engineered biological dressings. Tissue Eng 2006; 12(9):2407–24.

23. Falanga VJ. Tissue engineering in wound repair. Adv Skin Wound Care 2000;13(Suppl 2):15–9.

24. Falabella AF, Valencia IC, Eaglstein WH, et al. Tissue-engineered skin (Apligraf) in the healing of patients with epidermolysis bullosa wounds. Arch Dermatol 2000;136(10):1225–30.

25. Shores JT, Gabriel A, Gupta S. Skin substitutes and alternatives: a review. Adv Skin Wound Care 2007; 20(9 Pt 1):493–508 [quiz: 509–10].

26. Wood FM. Cultured human keratinocytes and tissue engineered skin substitutes. In: Horch RE, Munster AM,

Achauer BM, editors. Stuttgart (Germany): Thieme; 2001. p. 275–83.

27. Leigh IM, Purkis PE, Navsaria HA, et al. Treatment of chronic venous ulcers with sheets of cultured allogenic keratinocytes. Br J Dermatol 1987;117(5): 591–7.

28. De Luca M, Albanese E, Cancedda R, et al. Treatment of leg ulcers with cryopreserved allogeneic cultured epithelium. A multicenter study. Arch Dermatol 1992;128(5):633–8.

29. Haith LR Jr, Patton ML, Goldman WT. Cultured epidermal autograft and the treatment of the massive burn injury. J Burn Care Rehabil 1992;13(1):142–6.

30. Williamson JS, Snelling CF, Clugston P, et al. Cultured epithelial autograft: five years of clinical experience with twenty-eight patients. J Trauma 1995;39(2):309–19.

31. Wang TW, Wu HC, Huang YC, et al. Biomimetic bi-layered gelatin-chondroitin 6 sulfate-hyaluronic acid biopolymer as a scaffold for skin equivalent tissue engineering. Artif Organs 2006;30(3):141–9.

32. Navarro FA, Stoner ML, Park CS, et al. Sprayed keratinocyte suspensions accelerate epidermal coverage in a porcine microwound model. J Burn Care Rehabil 2000;21(6):513–8.

33. Fang RC, Galiano RD. A review of becaplermin gel in the treatment of diabetic neuropathic foot ulcers. Biologics 2008;2(1):1–12.

34. Bianco P, Riminucci M, Gronthos S, et al. Circulating skeletal stem cells: nature biology and potential applications. Stem Cells 2001;19:180–92.

35. Pittenger MF, Mackay AM, Beck SC, et al. Multilineage potential of adult human mesenchymal stem cells. Science 1999;284:143–7.

36. Falanga V, Iwamoto S, Chartier M, et al. Autologous bone marrow-derived cultured mesenchymal stem cells delivered in a fibrin spray accelerate healing in murine and human cutaneous wounds. Tissue Eng 2007;13(6):1299–312.

37. Badiavas EV, Falanaga V. Treatment of chronic wounds with bone marrow-derived cells. Arch Dermatol 2003;139:510–6.

38. Cha J, Falanga V. Stem cells in cutaneous wound healing. Clin Dermatol 2007;25(1):73–8.

39. Nataraj C, Ritter G, Dumas S, et al. Extracellular wound matrices: novel stabilization and sterilization method for collage-based biologic wound dressings. Wounds 2007;19(6):148–56.

40. Zheng MH, Chen J, Kirilak Y, et al. Porcine small intestine submucosa (SIS) is not an acellular matrix and contains porcine DNA: possible implications in human implantation. J Biomed Mater Res B Appl Biomater 2005;73(1):61–7.

41. Badylak SF, Gilbert TW. Immune response to biologic scaffold materials. Semin Immunol 2008;20(2): 109–16.

42. Mulder GD, Lee DK. Case presentation: xenograft resistance to protease degradation in a vasculitic ulcer. Int J Low Extrem Wounds 2009;8:157.

43. Powell HM, Boyce ST. EDC cross-linking improves skin substitute strength and stability. Biomaterials 2006;27(34):5821–7.

44. WU SC, Yoon H, Armstrong DG. Combining VAC therapy with advanced modalities: can it expedite healing? Podiatry Today 2005;18(9):18–24.

45. Niezgoda JA, Van Gills CC, Frykberg RG, et al. Randomized clinical trial comparing OASIS Wound Matrix to Regranex gel for diabetic ulcers. Adv Skin Wound Care 2005;18(5 Pt 1):258–66.

46. Brigido SA, Boc SF, Lopez RC. Effective management of major lower extremity wounds using an acellular regenerative tissue matrix: a pilot study. Orthopedics 2004;27(Suppl 1):s145–9.

47. Mulder GM, Lee DK. A retrospective clinical review of extracellular matrices for tissue reconstruction: equine pericardium as a biological covering to assist with wound closure. Wounds 2009;21(9):254–61.

48. Valentin JA, Bdjak JS, McCabe GP, et al. Extracellular matrix bioscaffolds for orthopaedic applications: a comparative histology study. J Bone Joint Surg Am 2006;88:2673–86.

Compression and Venous Surgery for Venous Leg Ulcers

Giovanni Mosti, MD

KEYWORDS

- Compression therapy • Elastic compression • Inelastic compression • Venous reflux
- Venous pumping function • Venous surgery

KEY POINTS

- Randomized controlled studies comparing surgery and compression point out that surgery and compression have similar effectiveness in producing ulcer healing but surgery is more effective in preventing recurrence.
- There is evidence that compression is better than no compression, compression with strong pressure is better than compression with mild to moderate pressure, and compression exerted by multi-component devices is better than compression by mono-component devices.
- Elastic stockings exerting the highest pressure that can be tolerated by the patient must be used after ulcer healing to prevent recurrence.

INTRODUCTION

In more than 70% of patients,[1,2] leg ulcers are caused by venous diseases, such as superficial or deep venous insufficiency and deep vein obstruction (**Fig. 1**). Venous reflux and reduced venous pumping function result in ambulatory venous hypertension (AVH).

The hydrostatic venous pressure in the lower leg in the standing position is about 70 to 80 mm Hg both in healthy individuals and in patients with venous disease, because it depends on the pressure exerted by the column of blood from the right heart to the ankle.

In the normal individual this pressure decreases significantly during active movement (eg, walking) because of venous pumping and the valvular function that fragments the blood column and reduces hydrostatic venous pressure.[3] In patients with venous insufficiency or obstruction, pressure decreases much less or may even increase because of reduced pumping function and valvular incompetence, and this condition is termed AVH.

The pathophysiological mechanisms leading from venous hypertension to skin changes and ulcer formation are still unclear and could be caused by varied mechanisms. Fibrin cuff formation around the microvessels, impaired exchange of gases (O_2, CO_2),[4] the entrapment of white cells[5] in the microvessels causing skin necrosis, and the inhibition of growth factors[6] causing stagnation of the healing process are responsible for skin break-down and delayed healing.

In the treatment of venous ulcers, the main aim is to counteract AVH, the most important cause of the skin damage. This is done by compression therapy, by elevating the leg, by walking, by the abolition of reflux by means of surgery (including ablation of superficial incompetent veins or perforator veins, catheter dilatation, and stenting or valve reconstruction of deep veins), or by more conservative methods, (endovascular procedures, such as laser therapy, radiofrequency ablation, foam sclerotherapy, or hemodynamic correction of venous insufficiency).

The author declares no conflict of interest.
Angiology Department, Clinica MD Barbantini, Via del Calcio 2, 5510 Lucca, Italy
E-mail address: jmosti@tin.it

Clin Plastic Surg 39 (2012) 269–280
doi:10.1016/j.cps.2012.04.004
0094-1298/12/$ – see front matter © 2012 Elsevier Inc. All rights reserved.

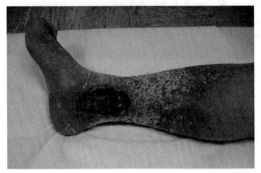

Fig. 1. Venous ulcers are typically located at the medial aspect of the leg in the supramalleolar area. Their size and ulcer bed condition are variable depending on ulcer duration and treatment. The peri-wound skin can be brown colored and is usually hard because of dermatosclerosis typical of venous insufficiency. Scaling is another typical feature of venous ulcers. Edema is present every time the ulcer is not treated by compression.

Compression therapy is able to narrow or occlude the leg veins[7] by applying appropriate external pressure to induce a valvular mechanism that reduces venous reflux[8,9] and increases the calf pumping function.[10]

The appropriate timing for compression and venous surgery and the choice of the compression most useful for the healing of ulcers, remain unclear (**Box 1**).

COMPRESSION OR VEIN SURGERY FOR ULCER HEALING

Several uncontrolled and nonrandomized studies have shown the beneficial effect of surgical procedures on venous ulcer healing.

Great saphenous vein crossectomy and stripping are claimed to improve venous function and heal leg venous ulcers without compression bandaging,

if the deep veins are normal. Compression is always necessary when a deep venous insufficiency coexists.[11,12]

Perforating vein interruption, sometimes associated with great saphenous vein stripping, has been performed to promote ulcer healing.[13–17] This procedure is reported to result in rapid ulcer healing, improvement in quality of life, and significant reduction of ulcer recurrence. Studies[13–17] conclude that "nihilism has no place in the management of venous disease in the 21st century",[14] that "surgery is indicated before an ulcer is intractable to treatment,"[14] and that "standard surgical methods can be applied for the therapy of venous leg ulcers at any stage."[17]

However, 2 different meta-analyses on compression therapy demonstrated significant effectiveness in ulcer healing.[18,19]

A prospective but not randomized study showed that, compared with compression, great saphenous vein surgery did not deliver better results in the ulcer healing rate; although a lower recurrence rate at 1–, 2–, and 3 years[20] was reported.

In controlled and randomized studies[21–23] the conclusions were similar[22]:

- Chronic venous leg ulceration was managed by compression treatment, elevation of the leg, and exercise
- Addition of ablative superficial venous surgery did not affect ulcer healing, but reduced ulcer recurrence.

In one study, the treatment of venous insufficiency by hemodynamic surgery was more effective than compression, both in healing and lowering the recurrence rate.[24]

In conclusion, there is almost general agreement that compression and surgery are equally effective in producing ulcer healing and improving quality of life; surgery is more effective than compression only in preventing ulcer recurrence.[25]

Endovascular procedures showed a beneficial effect in the ulcer healing process, in uncontrolled nonrandomized studies. However, no comparison with traditional surgery or compression proved the greater effectiveness of these procedures.[26–29]

Foam sclerotherapy was also used to speed the healing process in venous leg ulcers.[30–32] Foam in adjunct to compression, proved to be effective and demonstrated outcomes similar to surgery.[30,31] It seemed to accelerate the healing process.[32] Because foam sclerotherapy is almost always associated with compression therapy, studies comparing these 2 methods in ulcer healing do not exist (**Box 2**).

Box 1
Initial approach to leg ulcers

- Leg ulcers are frequently (in more than 70% of cases) caused by venous disease causing AVH.
- The first step to promote ulcer healing is to counteract AVH.
- This is done conservatively by compression therapy, by elevating the leg, by walking, or by ablating the vein by means of surgery, endovascular procedures, and foam sclerotherapy.

Box 2
Compression or vein surgery for ulcer healing

- Several uncontrolled and nonrandomized studies showed the beneficial effect of surgical procedures, such as great saphenous vein crossectomy and stripping and/or perforating vein interruption, on venous ulcer healing.

- Compared with compression, venous surgery did not reveal better results in the ulcer healing rate, but did reveal a lower recurrence rate at 1–, 2–, and 3 years.

- Uncontrolled, nonrandomized studies showed beneficial effect for endovascular procedures (laser and radiofrequency) and foam sclerotherapy in the ulcer healing process. Controlled randomized studies comparing these techniques with compression do not exist.

- There is an almost general agreement that compression and surgery are equally effective in ulcer healing and improving the quality of life; surgery is more effective than compression only in preventing ulcer recurrence.

CHOICE OF COMPRESSION IN THE TREATMENT OF ULCERS

The prerequisite for the effectiveness of compression on venous hemodynamics is a significant narrowing of the veins with short phases of intermittent occlusion during walking to prevent venous reflux, increase the venous ejection fraction and reduce AVH.

To narrow or occlude the venous system, the compression pressure must be higher than the intravenous pressure. This depends on the body position because venous pressure varies in different body positions. It has been shown that it is possible to narrow or occlude the veins with an external pressure of 20 mm Hg in the supine position, 50 mm Hg in the sitting position, and 70 mm Hg in the standing position.[33] It was also demonstrated that in the sitting position a pressure of 40 mm Hg was enough to narrow (but not occlude) the calf veins; but when the patient was asked to do foot dorsiflexions with an inelastic cuff, the pressure increased to 60 mm Hg, resulting in vein occlusion. These data were confirmed by magnetic resonance imaging studies, which showed that in the standing position, a pressure of 40 mm Hg was not able to occlude the veins, that were only completely occluded with a pressure of 80 mm Hg (**Fig. 2**).[7]

In conclusion standing venous pressure can be modified by an external compression pressure higher than 60 mm Hg (defined as very strong in a recent consensus paper).[34]

Compression materials are classified into elastic and inelastic categories. Both categories exert pressure on the leg that depends on the stretch applied to the bandage, the number of turns in the bandage, and the radius of the leg segment (Laplace law).[35]

An intelligent compression system should exert a very strong pressure in the standing position and a low and comfortable resting pressure in the supine position. It should have a large difference between standing and resting pressure. This difference has been termed Static Stiffness

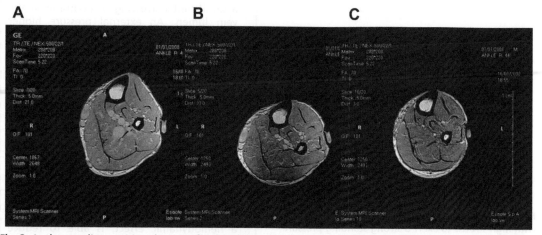

A **B** **C**

Fig. 2. In the standing position the superficial and deep leg veins are significantly dilated (*A*). An elastic stocking exerting a standing position of 38 mm Hg has no effect on the superficial veins whereas it occludes the muscle veins (*B*); an inelastic bandage exerting a pressure of 81 mm Hg occludes both superficial and deep veins (*C*).

Index (SSI) and it is one of the most important indicators of the stiffness of the bandage.[36,37] Elastic material gives way to muscle expansion that results in a very low difference between the resting pressure and the pressure in standing position or during functional activities. For elastic material, the SSI is usually less than 10 mm Hg. During muscular activity, the difference between systolic and diastolic pressure termed walking pressure amplitude (WPA), another indicator of the stiffness of the bandage, is very low.

In addition elastic material tends to return to its original length when extended and its return power is directly related to the stretch applied to the bandage (squeezing effect). As a consequence, in order to produce the strong standing pressure necessary to counteract AVH, an elastic bandage must be applied at full stretch. This application method exerts a very strong pressure also in the supine position (**Fig. 3**). The resulting bandage will be painful and intolerable to the patient and should be avoided in the clinical setting.

An elastic bandage should be applied at 50% of its total extensibility to avoid being painful. In this condition the supine pressure is not higher than 40 to 45 mm Hg, resulting in a standing pressure not higher than 45 to 50 mm Hg, which is not enough to occlude the veins (**Fig. 4**).

An inelastic bandage, made up of a short stretch of inextensible material, exerts its effect by resisting the increase of muscle volume during muscular contraction in the upright position and during functional activities (the leg gives way) and it does not exert any elastic return effect.

Inelastic bandages are well tolerated at rest even when applied with strong initial pressure, because the leg volume reduces immediately due to the reduction of physiological oedema,

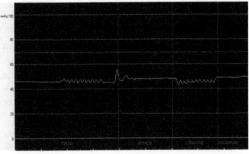

Fig. 4. Pressure curve of an elastic bandage correctly applied; the supine pressure is 43 mm Hg resulting in a standing pressure of 46 mm Hg that is not enough to occlude the veins.

resulting in a very fast pressure loss into a tolerable range. At the same time, it exerts a much higher pressure during standing (SSI always >10) and strong or very strong pressure peaks during muscular exercise, higher than 70 mm Hg, enough to intermittently occlude the veins and restore a kind of valvular mechanism starting from a fairly low and tolerable resting pressure. For these reasons the inelastic bandage system comes close to the criteria for an ideal compression system (**Box 3**, **Fig. 5**).[38]

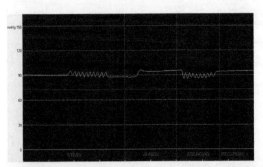

Fig. 3. Pressure curve of an elastic bandage applied with high stretch to exert a strong standing pressure. The supine pressure must be strong to guarantee a strong standing pressure. This sustained pressure can be painful.

Box 3
Choice of compression material for treatment of venous ulcers

- The pre-requisite for the effectiveness of compression on venous hemodynamics is a significant narrowing or occlusion of the vein lumen. An external pressure higher than 60 mm Hg is necessary in the standing position to occlude the veins.

- Compression materials are classified into elastic and inelastic materials.

- Elastic material is not able to achieve strong pressure in the standing position when properly applied.

- Inelastic material exerts a very high standing pressure and strong or very strong pressure peaks during muscular exercise. This pressure is able to intermittently occlude the venous lumen.

- For these reasons the inelastic bandage has a hemodynamic effect, is able to reduce AVH and should be preferred in ulcer treatment.

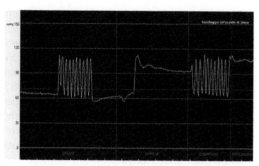

Fig. 5. Pressure curve of an inelastic bandage. It can be applied with full stretch exerting a supine pressure of 60 mm Hg, not painful because the material has no elastic return. The standing or working pressure is easily more than 70 mm Hg (the venous pressure in the leg in the standing position), restoring a kind of valvular function.

THE PRACTICAL CONSEQUENCES OF DIFFERENT COMPRESSION PRESSURE PROFILES ON VENOUS REFLUX AND IMPAIRED VENOUS PUMPING FUNCTION
Effect on Venous Reflux

Inelastic material is more effective than elastic material in reducing venous reflux in venous insufficiency. In a previous study,[9] in patients with deep venous insufficiency, the air plethysmographic parameters venous volume (VV) and venous filling index (VFI) were reduced by increasing external pressure; the reduction was significantly greater with inelastic than with elastic compression materials because the former achieved a much higher standing pressure starting from the same supine pressure. The investigators concluded that, "using the same bandage pressure, inelastic compression material is more effective at reducing deep venous refluxes than elastic bandages, in patients with venous ulcers."

In a more recent work we came to the same conclusion in patients affected by superficial venous insufficiency, by measuring the reflux volume automatically calculated by the Duplex scanner.[8]

Twelve patients were examined in the standing position by means of the Duplex scanner Esaote Mylab 60 (Esaote, Florence, Italy) with a specially designed finger-like probe (Esaote IOE323 Intraoperative, Linear Array 4–13 MHz) without any compression and after the application of different compression devices from the base of the toes to the knee. This probe finger-like 12 MHz probe was fixed with tapes at the mid-thigh, on the incompetent GSV along the longitudinal axis and its position was never changed during the experiments. The reflux was elicited by tip-toe maneuvers and measured when the patient returned to the upright relaxed position after tip-toeing. After recording the baseline measurements without any compression, the authors applied elastic and inelastic devices at the same supine pressure of 20–, 40–, and 60 mm Hg. The resulting standing pressures were significantly higher with inelastic material compared with elastic and inelastic material resulted in significantly higher reduction of venous reflux. Only when the authors applied elastic bandages with 60 mm Hg pressure, the reflux was reduced to an extent similar to inelastic compression, but this high pressure was intolerable to the patient and was used only for the short duration of the laboratory test and not in daily practice.

Effect on Venous Pumping Function

Inelastic material is more effective than elastic material in improving venous pumping function that is severely reduced in venous insufficiency. In different experiments conducted on 68 patients affected by major reflux in the great saphenous vein (CEAP C3-C5 classification), the authors measured the ejection fraction (EF) of the venous calf pump by means of strain gauge plethysmography[10,39–41] according to a previously described protocol (Poelkens and colleagues).[42] The investigation started with leg elevation to empty the veins. The minimal volume of the leg segment proximal to the bandage was registered by the strain gauge. Then the patient stood up and the volume increase of the calf segment that reflected venous filling, was measured continuously. Venous volume (VV) is defined as the difference between empty and filled veins. During a standardized exercise (20 steps on a 20 cm high stair in 20 seconds) the volume of blood that is expelled toward the heart (EV) reflects the quality of the venous pump. The proportion of EV in relation to VV expressed as a percentage, is the EF (**Box 4**).

Box 4
Effects of elastic and inelastic compression materials on the venous pumping function

- Compared with elastic material, inelastic material is more effective in reducing venous reflux and increasing the venous pumping function in patients with superficial and deep venous insufficiency.

- These effects occur independently from the pressure at application and even at a low pressure of 20 mm Hg.

- Inelastic material maintains its positive effect up to 1 week despite a significant drop in pressure over time.

After the baseline measurements without any compression, the authors applied compression with elastic and inelastic materials at the same pressures of 20–, 40–, and 60 mm Hg. After patients stood up, the pressures increased significantly with the use of inelastic material compared with elastic material, and the EF increased slightly but significantly with elastic material and was restored to the normal range only by the inelastic material (**Table 1**).[10,39]

In these series of experiments 3 findings were noteworthy:

1. Elastic material does not improve the venous pumping function at the same extent as inelastic material, not even when applied with maximal stretch to exert a standing pressure of 60 mm Hg. Despite this high pressure, the increase of EF was always modest and significantly lower than the improvement achieved by inelastic material. Furthermore, this pressure was hard for the patient to tolerate and was applied only for short durations. The EF improvement showed significant correlation with the standing pressure, the pressure differences during movement (massaging effect), and especially with the pressure peaks (working pressure).[10]
2. This significant superiority of inelastic material was also seen at a very low pressure of 20 mm Hg. At this pressure the elastic material barely showed a hemodynamic effect, whereas inelastic material increased the EF values almost into the normal range.[40] This finding has significance in the use of inelastic compression systems with reduced pressure in the treatment of mixed arterio-venous ulcers.
3. Despite a significant pressure drop, the effect of inelastic material was maintained over time. The authors measured the EF not only immediately after elastic and inelastic bandage application but also after 7 days of wearing time.

Table 1
Percentage improvement in EF increase with elastic and inelastic material applied with different pressures

	20 mm Hg	40 mm Hg	60 mm Hg
Elastic material	+19%	+32%	+37%
Inelastic material	+63%	+83%	+86%

Data from Mosti G, Partsch H. Measuring venous pumping function by strain-gauge plethysmography. Int Angiol 2010;29(5):421–5.

They observed that the pressure of inelastic material dropped significantly, whereas with the elastic material the pressure drop was much less. Nevertheless, the stiffness and the efficacy of the inelastic bandage was maintained over time as demonstrated by high SSI and WPA (that were substantially unchanged after 1 week) and EF remained still in the normal range. The effect of elastic material, which was poor immediately after application, continued to be poor after 7 days.[41]

INELASTIC COMPRESSION AND MIXED LEG ULCERS

About 15% to 20% of patients with venous leg ulcers have arterial impairments that cause retarded healing. In these patients, compression improves venous hemodynamics but could impair arterial inflow.

In 25 patients (10 men, 15 women), aged 76 years,(± 4 to 10 years) with mixed ulcers presenting a mean ankle brachial pressure index (ABPI) value of 0.57(± 0.09), the authors tried to define a range of compression pressures that did not impede arterial flow but was still able to improve the venous pumping function.[43] The skin flow in the peri-wound area and in the plantar surface of the first toe and toe pressure were assessed by means of laser doppler flowmetry. Trancutaneous oxygen pressure on the foot dorsum distal to the bandage was measured. The measurements were taken in baseline conditions and after inelastic bandages were applied with pressure ranges of 20 to 30 mm Hg, 30 to 40 mm Hg, and 40 to 50 mm Hg. Bandage pressure was continuously measured by a pneumatic device. The venous pumping function was assessed by strain gauge plethysmography measuring the EF from the lower leg in baseline conditions and after application of reduced compression.

Skin perfusion around the ulcer increased significantly with bandage pressures of 20 to 30 mm Hg and 30 to 40 mm Hg and returned to the baseline level with a bandage pressure of 40 to 50 mm Hg (**Fig. 6**A). Toe perfusion showed minor insignificant decrease with bandage pressures of 20 to 30 mm Hg and 30 to 40 mm Hg but registered significant reduction with 40 to 50 mm Hg pressure. Toe pressure increased with every pressure step, showing significant differences compared with baseline values with bandage pressures of 30 to 40 mm Hg and 40 to 50 mm Hg (see **Fig. 6**B). EF increased significantly with a bandage pressure of 20 to 30 mm Hg and was restored to the normal range with bandage pressure of 30 to 40 mm Hg (see **Fig. 6**C).

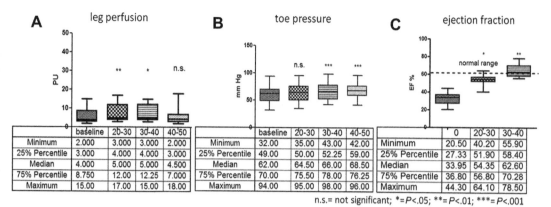

	baseline	20-30	30-40	40-50
Minimum	2.000	3.000	3.000	2.000
25% Percentile	3.000	4.000	4.000	3.000
Median	4.000	5.000	5.000	4.500
75% Percentile	8.750	12.00	12.25	7.000
Maximum	15.00	17.00	15.00	18.00

	baseline	20-30	30-40	40-50
Minimum	32.00	35.00	43.00	42.00
25% Percentile	49.00	50.00	52.25	59.00
Median	62.00	64.50	66.00	68.50
75% Percentile	70.00	75.50	78.00	76.25
Maximum	94.00	95.00	98.00	96.00

	0	20-30	30-40
Minimum	20.50	40.20	55.90
25% Percentile	27.33	51.90	58.40
Median	33.95	54.35	62.60
75% Percentile	36.80	56.80	70.28
Maximum	44.30	64.10	78.50

n.s.= not significant; *=$P<.05$; **=$P<.01$; ***=$P<.001$

Fig. 6. In mixed ulcers skin perfusion increases significantly with bandage pressures of 20–30 mm Hg and 30–40 mm Hg and start to decrease with 40–50 mm Hg (A). Toe pressure increases with every pressure step (B). EF increases significantly with a bandage pressure 20–30 mm Hg and is restored into the normal range with 30–40 mm Hg (C).

In conclusion, external compression up to 40 mm Hg significantly increased arterial flow, (even in patients with very low ABPI values and venous EF) and may be considered the basic treatment modality in managing patients with mixed ulceration.

In this experiment the authors avoided elastic material because elastic return power could be painful for patients with reduced arterial inflow, even when applied with low compression pressure. In addition, they took advantage of the hemodynamic superiority of inelastic bandages demonstrated in their previous studies (**Box 5**).[10]

ELASTIC OR INELASTIC BANDAGES FOR PATIENTS WITH LEG ULCERS AND RESTRICTED MOBILITY?

Some old textbooks claim that inelastic material only works during exercise and is therefore ineffective for patients with restricted or absent mobility of the ankle joint. If a patient is completely immobile and bedridden, a simple antiembolic stocking exerting a pressure of about 20 mm Hg

is enough to narrow the veins. But if the patient is able to move some steps and sit in a chair, a pressure of 50 mm Hg is necessary to influence the vein lumen in the sitting position and 70 mm Hg in the standing position. Elastic material is not able to exert this strong or very strong pressure. Moreover simple ankle movements either active or induced by a physiotherapist, produce intermittent peaks (massaging effect), which are much higher with an inelastic bandage than with an elastic bandage (**Fig. 7**) and result in a stronger effect on the venous pumping function. Daily experience shows that wheelchair-bound patients presenting with swelling and leg ulceration benefit dramatically from inelastic bandages, which may stay on the leg for several days and nights, needing to be changed only when they become very loose.[44,45]

Relationship between Hemodynamic Efficacy and Ulcer Healing Rate

When inelastic bandages are correctly applied and the intended pressure is achieved, the outcomes on venous ulcers can be spectacular with a healing rate close to 100%, as shown in a recent trial[46] that compared 2 inelastic bandage systems used in the treatment of venous ulcers. In this trial, both compression systems were applied with pressures higher than 40 mm Hg. Pressure was measured at bandage application to ensure that the correct pressure range was applied with both systems and also measured at bandage removal to check the bandage pressure loss. Because of the strong pressure at application and the maintenance of high SSI values over time, all the patients except one (who withdrew because of an ulcer infection) healed in both compression groups and 92 out of 99 patients healed within 3 months.

Box 5
Inelastic compression for mixed leg ulcers

- Inelastic material with a reduced pressure of 30 to 40 mm Hg was safely used in patients with mixed ulcerations without affecting and even improving the arterial inflow.

- Inelastic material showed a better effect on pressure amplitude and, as a consequence, on reflux and pumping function, and also in patients with reduced mobility.

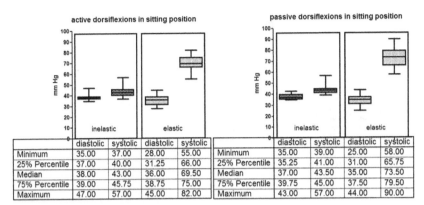

| active dorsiflexions in sitting position | | | | | passive dorsiflexions in sitting position | | | | |
	diastolic	systolic	diastolic	systolic		diastolic	systolic	diastolic	systolic
Minimum	35.00	37.00	28.00	55.00	Minimum	35.00	39.00	25.00	58.00
25% Percentile	37.00	40.00	31.25	66.00	25% Percentile	35.25	41.00	31.00	65.75
Median	38.00	43.00	36.00	69.50	Median	37.00	43.50	35.00	73.50
75% Percentile	39.00	45.75	38.75	75.00	75% Percentile	39.75	45.00	37.50	79.50
Maximum	47.00	57.00	45.00	82.00	Maximum	43.00	57.00	44.00	90.00

Fig. 7. Active (*left side*) and passive (*right side*) dorsiflections in a patient with reduced mobility in sitting position. Inelastic material produces much higher pressure peaks starting from similar diastolic values both in active and passive exercise.

Many investigators have claimed the superiority of elastic material (both elastic stockings and elastic bandages) compared with inelastic material. This contradicts all the reported data showing more favourable hemodynamic effects for inelastic material.

Unfortunately the clinical studies reporting the superiority of elastic material have major flaws.

Limitations of Studies of Elastic and Inelastic Bandages

1. The pressure exerted by compression devices was almost never measured in studies comparing different compression devices, although compression pressure is considered the "dosage" of compression and the main determinant of its effect. When the compression pressure produced by a compression device is not measured, there is no information on the principal determinant of its effectiveness. Furthermore, when compression pressure is not measured, it is difficult to determine if bandages were correctly applied, if the intended pressure for a specific bandage was achieved, and if the exerted pressure is consistent in different centers or in different bandages applied by the same bandager. The absence of sub-bandage pressure measurements in older studies was caused by the lack of effective, simple, inexpensive, and reproducible measurement devices. This is no longer the case and such devices are now available.[47,48] They were used in all the author's investigations.

2. In the published articles comparing elastic and inelastic bandages,[49–51] the prototype of the elastic material was Profore® (Smith and Nephew, UK), which works like an inelastic bandage. Profore® is made up of 4 different mainly elastic components but the overlapping of different textiles changes the elastic properties of the final bandage, especially because of the friction between the layers. This may explain why Profore® has an SSI that is close to the Rosidal sys® (Lohmann Rausscher, Germany) bandage that is mainly composed of inelastic textiles.[52]

3. In effect, all the studies report comparison between 2 different inelastic bandages and not between an elastic and an inelastic bandage. It is possible that the "different" but actually very similar compression devices had similar results.

4. The so-called elastic material may have delivered the best outcomes because of the better expertise of the bandagers applying this compression device (**Box 6**).

COMPARISON BETWEEN ELASTIC STOCKINGS AND INELASTIC BANDAGES

A recent meta-analysis reported that "leg compression with stockings is clearly better than compression with bandages, has a positive impact on pain, and is easier to use."[53] Unfortunately this meta-analysis contains errors in the reporting of some quoted studies (**Box 7**).

1. The elastic stockings used for comparison were actually elastic kits or tubular devices exerting a high supine pressure of 40 mm Hg or more and higher stiffness (although always in the recommended range of stiffness for elastic material), because of the friction between 2 components.[54–58]

2. Neither sub-bandage pressure measurements nor bandagers' skills in applying the inelastic bandage were reported. Without pressure

Box 6
Comparison of elastic and inelastic bandages on venous ulcer outcomes

- When correctly applied and the intended pressure achieved, the outcomes of inelastic bandages on venous ulcers are extremely positive (healing rate close to 100%).
- Studies claiming the superiority of elastic material (both elastic stockings and elastic bandages) compared with inelastic materials were almost always performed without measuring the pressure of the compression devices.
- Pressure represents the "dosage" of compression and when not measured, make the results of these studies unreliable.
- The bandage almost always used as the elastic comparision in these studies is actually inelastic.

measurements, only the pressure of elastic kits as declred by the manufacturer was available and there was no information on the pressure of the inelastic bandage, which can be

Box 7
Comparison of elastic stockings with inelastic materials

- A meta-analysis reporting the comparison between elastic stockings and inelastic material has some errors.
- The elastic stockings taken into consideration for comparison were actually elastic kits or tubular devices exerting a high supine pressure of 40 mm Hg or more with greater stiffness.
- Neither sub-bandage pressure measurements nor bandagers' skills in applying the inelastic bandage have been reported.
- In one study the patients or their relatives were even allowed to remove the bandage in the evening and reapply it on the following morning.
- In a few studies that measured compression pressure, it was demonstrated that the higher the pressure of the bandage, the higher was the healing rate. This conclusion is clearly in favor of bandages that, when correctly applied, exert a compression pressure definitely higher than elastic stockings or kits.
- Elastic stockings exerting the highest pressure tolerable to the patients, should be used after ulcer healing to prevent recurrence.

extremely variable[59–61] because it is wholly dependent on the stretch applied to the bandage by the bandager. In one study, the patients were even allowed to remove the bandage in the evening and re-apply it on the following morning.[55] The variability of bandage pressure is high even when the bandages are applied by expert doctors and nurses and it is conceivable that variability is even higher when patients or relatives reapply the bandage.

All these elements make it difficult to understand if the bandages were correctly applied and certainly a good elastic kit could work better than a poorly applied bandage (both elastic and inelastic). In a few studies (some of them also referenced in the meta-analysis) that measured compression pressure,[57,58,62,63] it was demonstrated that the higher the pressure applied the higher was the healing rate. This conclusion is clearly in favor of bandages that, when correctly applied, exert a compression pressure definitely higher than elastic stockings or kits.

COMPRESSION AFTER ULCER HEALING

After ulcer healing, compression must be continued to prevent ulcer recurrence. This is the best indication for elastic stockings. Because the higher the compression pressure applied the lower is the recurrence rate, the highest pressure tolerated by the patients is recommended.[64]

SUMMARY

- Treatment of leg ulcers must be based first on the correction of hemodynamic impairment. This can be done conservatively by means of compression, walking and leg elevation, or by surgical removal of venous reflux.
- To achieve the best results, compression therapy must be correctly applied. It should exert a high pressure in standing and working conditions to counteract venous hemodynamic impairment (venous reflux, reduced venous pumping function), starting from a lower and tolerable supine pressure.
- Venous surgery has been shown to be as effective as compression therapy in promoting ulcer healing and improving quality of life. Surgery is more effective than compression in preventing ulcer recurrence. Many surgical procedures have been proposed, from crossectomy and stripping to perforator interruption and endovascular procedures (laser, radiofrequency). More conservative procedures to abolish venous

reflux (foam sclerotherapy, conservative hemodynamic treatment) have also been proposed in ulcer treatment.

- There is convincing evidence that inelastic compression material is more effective than elastic compression material in reducing venous reflux and in improving the venous pumping function and that it is more tolerable at rest. Inelastic material is more effective at every pressure range (mild, medium and strong) and is effective over time. It is more effective even in patients with reduced mobility and it is able to improve (rather than decrease) the sub-bandage and periwound flux in patients with arterial impairment, if applied with reduced pressure. There is proof that inelastic material, applied with the same initial pressure, is significantly more effective than elastic material in improving the hemodynamic impairment of venous insufficiency. This results in the higher effectiveness of inelastic material in promoting ulcer healing, when properly applied.
- The so-called multilayer bandages consisting of several elastic components are in the end, stiff because of the friction between the layers, so that the designation "elastic" is inadequate. The "elastic" bandage very often considered as the material for comparison in these studies is actually an inelastic bandage, making the comparison inconsistent with the aim of the studies.
- Clear clinical evidence confirming the superiority of inelastic bandages compared with elastic bandages in promoting ulcer healing is lacking because of major flaws reported in the clinical studies.
- A multicentre randomized study, with experienced bandagers and sub-bandage pressure measurements to ensure the correct application of the bandage and achieve the intended pressure range, is highly recommended

REFERENCES

1. Adam DJ, Naik J, Hartshorne T, et al. The diagnosis and management of 689 chronic leg ulcers in a single-visit assessment clinic. Eur J Vasc Endovasc Surg 2003;25(5):462–8.
2. Baker SR, Stacey MC, Singh G, et al. Aetiology of chronic leg ulcers. Eur J Vasc Surg 1992;6(3):245–51.
3. Arnoldi CC. Venous pressure in the leg of healthy human subjects at rest and during muscular exercise in the nearly erect position. Acta Chir Scand 1965;130(6):570–83.
4. Browse NL, Burnand KG. The cause of venous ulceration. Lancet 1982;2(8292):243–5.
5. Coleridge Smith PD, Thomas P, Scurr JH, et al. Causes of venous ulceration: a new hypothesis. Br Med J (Clin Res Ed) 1988;296(6638):1726–7.
6. Falanga V, Eaglstein WH. The "trap" hypothesis of venous ulceration. Lancet 1993;341(8851):1006–8.
7. Partsch H, Mosti G, Mosti F. Narrowing of leg veins under compression demonstrated by magnetic resonance imaging (MRI). Int Angiol 2010;29(5):408–10.
8. Mosti G, Partsch H. Duplex scanning to evaluate the effect of compression on venous reflux. Int Angiol 2010;29(5):416–20.
9. Partsch H, Menzinger G, Mostbeck A. Inelastic leg compression is more effective to reduce deep venous refluxes than elastic bandages. Dermatol Surg 1999;25(9):695–700.
10. Mosti G, Mattaliano V, Partsch H. Inelastic compression increases venous ejection fraction more than elastic bandages in patients with superficial venous reflux. Phlebology 2008;23(6):287–94.
11. Scriven JM, Hartshorne T, Thrush AJ, et al. Role of saphenous vein surgery in the treatment of venous ulceration. Br J Surg 1998;85(6):781–4.
12. Bello M, Scriven JM, Hartshorne T, et al. Role of saphenous vein surgery in the treatment of venous ulceration. Br J Surg 1999;86(6):755–9.
13. Gloviczki P, Bergan JJ, Rhodes JM, et al. Mid-term results of endoscopic perforator vein interruption for chronic venous insufficiency: lessons learned from the North American subfascial endoscopic perforator surgery registry. The North American Study Group. J Vasc Surg 1999;29(3):489–502.
14. Iafrati MD, Pare GJ, O'Donnell TF, et al. Is the nihilistic approach to surgical reduction of superficial and perforator vein incompetence for venous ulcer justified? J Vasc Surg 2002;36(6):1167–74.
15. Roka F, Binder M, Bohler-Sommeregger K. Mid-term recurrence rate of incompetent perforating veins after combined superficial vein surgery and subfascial endoscopic perforating vein surgery. J Vasc Surg 2006;44(2):359–63.
16. Nelzén O, Fransson I. True long-term healing and recurrence of venous leg ulcers following SEPS combined with superficial venous surgery: a prospective study. Eur J Vasc Endovasc Surg 2007;34(5):605–12.
17. Obermayer A, Göstl K, Walli G, et al. Chronic venous leg ulcers benefit from surgery: long-term results from 173 legs. J Vasc Surg 2006;44(3):572–9.
18. Cullum N, Nelson EA, Fletcher AW, et al. Compression for venous leg ulcers. Cochrane Database Syst Rev 2001;2:CD000265.
19. Partsch H. Evidence based compression therapy. VASA 2003;32(Suppl 63):3–39.

20. Barwell JR, Taylor M, Deacon J, et al. Surgical correction of isolated superficial venous reflux reduces long-term recurrence rate in chronic venous leg ulcers. Eur J Vasc Endovasc Surg 2000;20(4): 363–8.

21. Guest M, Smith JJ, Tripuraneni G, et al. Randomized clinical trial of varicose vein surgery with compression versus compression alone for the treatment of venous ulceration. Phlebology 2003;18:130–6.

22. Barwell JR, Davies CE, Deacon J, et al. Comparison of surgery and compression with compression alone in chronic venous ulceration (ESCHAR study): randomised controlled trial. Lancet 2004;363(9424): 1854–9.

23. van Gent WB, Hop WC, van Praag MC, et al. Conservative versus surgical treatment of venous leg ulcers: a prospective, randomized, multicenter trial. J Vasc Surg 2006;44(3):563–71.

24. Zamboni P, Cisno C, Marchetti F, et al. Minimally invasive surgical management of primary venous ulcers vs. compression treatment: a randomised clinical trial. Eur J Vasc Endovasc Surg 2003;25(4):313–8.

25. Howard DP, Howard A, Kothari A, et al. The role of superficial venous surgery in the management of venous ulcers: a systematic review. Eur J Vasc Endovasc Surg 2008;36(4):458–65.

26. Sufian S, Lakhanpal S, Marquez J. Superficial vein ablation for the treatment of primary chronic venous ulcers. Phlebology 2011;26(7):301–6.

27. Teo TK, Tay KH, Lin SE, et al. Endovenous laser therapy in the treatment of lower-limb venous ulcers. J Vasc Interv Radiol 2010;21(5):657–62.

28. Sharif MA, Lau LL, Lee B, et al. Role of endovenous laser treatment in the management of chronic venous insufficiency. Ann Vasc Surg 2007;21(5):551–5.

29. Marrocco CJ, Atkins MD, Bohannon WT, et al. Endovenous ablation for the treatment of chronic venous insufficiency and venous ulcerations. World J Surg 2010;34(10):2299–304.

30. Pang KH, Bate GR, Darvall KA, et al. Healing and recurrence rates following ultrasound-guided foam sclerotherapy of superficial venous reflux in patients with chronic venous ulceration. Eur J Vasc Endovasc Surg 2010;40(6):790–5.

31. Darvall KA, Bate GR, Adam DJ, et al. Ultrasound-guided foam sclerotherapy for the treatment of chronic venous ulceration: a preliminary study. Eur J Vasc Endovasc Surg 2009;38(6):764–9.

32. O'Hare JL, Earnshaw JJ. Randomised clinical trial of foam sclerotherapy for patients with a venous leg ulcer. Eur J Vasc Endovasc Surg 2010;39(4):495–9.

33. Partsch B, Partsch H. Calf compression pressure required to achieve venous closure from supine to standing positions. J Vasc Surg 2005;42:734–8.

34. Partsch H, Clark M, Mosti G, et al. Classification of compression bandages: practical aspects. Dermatol Surg 2008;34:600–9.

35. Thomas S. The use of the Laplace equation in the calculation of sub-bandage pressure. EWMA J 2003;1:21–3.

36. Partsch H. The static stiffness index: a simple method to assess the elastic property of compression material in vivo. Dermatol Surg 2005;31: 625–30.

37. Partsch H. The use of pressure change on standing as a surrogate measure of the stiffness of a compression bandage. Eur J Vasc Endovasc Surg 2005;30: 415–21.

38. Partsch H. Compression therapy of venous ulcers. EWMA J 2006;2:16–20.

39. Mosti G, Partsch H. Measuring venous pumping function by strain-gauge plethysmography. Int Angiol 2010;29(5):421–5.

40. Mosti G, Partsch H. Is low compression pressure able to improve venous pumping function in patients with venous insufficiency? Phlebology 2010;25(3): 145–50.

41. Mosti G, Partsch H. Inelastic bandages maintain their hemodynamic effectiveness over time despite significant pressure loss. J Vasc Surg 2010;52(4): 925–31.

42. Poelkens F, Thijssen DH, Kersten B, et al. Counteracting venous stasis during acute lower leg immobilization. Acta Physiol (Oxf) 2006;186(2):111–8.

43. Mosti G, Iabichella ML, Partsch H. Compression therapy in mixed ulcers increases venous output and arterial perfusion. J Vasc Surg 2012;55(1): 122–8.

44. Mosti G. La terapia compressiva nel paziente con lesioni trofiche degli arti inferiori immobile o con mobilità limitata. Acta Vulnologica 2009;7(4):197–205 [in Italian].

45. Partsch H. Quelle compression sur des patients immobiles: allongement court ou allongement long? Geriatrie et Gerontologie 2009;155:278–83 [in French].

46. Mosti G, Crespi A, Mattaliano V. Comparison between a new, two-component compression system with zinc paste bandages for leg ulcer healing: a prospective, multicenter, randomized, controlled trial monitoring sub-bandage pressures. Wounds 2011;23(5):126–34.

47. Mosti G, Rossari S. L'importanza della misurazione della pressione sottobendaggio e presentazione di un nuovo strumento di misura. Acta Vulnol 2008;6: 31–6 [in Italian].

48. Partsch H, Mosti G. Comparison of three portable instruments to measure compression pressure. Int Angiol 2010;29(5):426–30.

49. Franks PJ, Moody M, Moffatt CJ, et al. Randomised trial of cohesive short-stretch versus four-layer bandaging in the management of venous ulceration. Wound Repair Regen 2004;12:157–62.

50. Callam MJ, Harper DR, Dale JJ, et al. Lothian Forth Valley leg ulcer healing trial—part 1: elastic versus

non-elastic bandaging in the treatment of chronic leg ulceration. Phlebology 1992;7:136–41.

51. Duby T, Hofman D, Cameron J, et al. A randomized trial in the treatment of venous leg ulcers comparing short stretch bandages, four layer bandage system, and a long stretch-paste bandage system. Wounds 1993;5:276–9.

52. Mosti G, Mattaliano V, Partsch H. Influence of different materials in multicomponent bandages on pressure and stiffness of the final bandage. Dermatol Surg 2008;34:631–9.

53. Amsler F, Willenberg T, Blättler W. Management of venous ulcer: a meta analysis of randomized studies comparing bandages to specifically designed stockings. J Vasc Surg 2009;50:668–74.

54. Mariani F, Mattaliano V, Mosti G, et al. The treatment of venous leg ulcers with a specifically designed compression stocking kit. Phlebologie 2008;37: 191–7.

55. Junger M, Partsch H, Ramelet AA, et al. Efficacy of a ready-made tubular compression device versus short stretch bandages in the treatment of venous leg ulcers. Wounds 2004;16:313–20.

56. Jünger M, Wollina U, Kohnen R, et al. Efficacy and tolerability of an ulcer compression stocking for therapy of chronic venous ulcer compared with a below-knee compression bandage: results from a prospective, randomized, multicentre trial. Curr Med Res Opin 2004;20(10):1613–23.

57. Horakova MA, Partsch H. Compression stockings in treatment of lower leg venous ulcer. Wien Med Wochenschr 1994;144(10–11):242–9.

58. Brizzio E, Amsler F, Lun B, et al. Comparison of low-strength compression stockings with bandages for the treatment of recalcitrant venous ulcers. J Vasc Surg 2010;51:410–6.

59. Partsch H. Variability of interface pressure exerted by compression bandages and standard size compression stockings. Proceedings of 20th Annual Meeting of American Venous Forum. Charleston (SC), February 20–23, 2008.

60. Moffat C. Variability of pressure provided by sustained compression. Int Wound J 2008;5(2):259–65.

61. Keller A, Müller ML, Calow T, et al. Bandage pressure measurement and training: simple interventions to improve efficacy in compression bandaging. Int Wound J 2009;6(5):324–30.

62. Milic DJ, Zivic SS, Bogdanovic DC, et al. A randomized trial of the Tubulcus multilayer bandaging system in the treatment of extensive venous ulcers. J Vasc Surg 2007;46:750–5.

63. Milic DJ, Zivic SS, Bogdanovic DC, et al. The influence of different sub-bandage pressure values on venous leg ulcers healing when treated with compression therapy. J Vasc Surg 2010;51(3):655–61.

64. Nelson EA, Bell-Syer SE, Cullum NA. Compression for preventing recurrence of venous ulcers. Cochrane Database Syst Rev 2000;4:CD002303.

Early Experiences with Stem Cells in Treating Chronic Wounds

Sadanori Akita, MD, PhD[a],*, Hiroshi Yoshimoto, MD, PhD[a],
Kozo Akino, MD, PhD[a], Akira Ohtsuru, MD, PhD[b,c],
Kenji Hayashida, MD, PhD[a], Akiyoshi Hirano, MD[a],
Keiji Suzuki, PhD[d], Shunichi Yamashita, MD, PhD[b,c,d]

KEYWORDS

- Nagasaki - Clinical study - Adipose-derived stem cell therapy for local chronic radiation injury

KEY POINTS

- Stem cell biology and application in wound healing is widely studied for bone marrow-derived stem cells.
- Adipose-derived stem cells (ADSCs) are more easily obtained from the donor sites.
- In chronic radiation injury, a mixture of ADSC and aspirated adipose tissue may play a pivotal role in wound healing.

INTRODUCTION
Wound Healing Process

The wound healing process contains well-organized and integrated patterns of complex biologic, molecular, and gene involvement events of

- Cell proliferation
- Cell migration
- Differentiation capacity of cells
- Extracellular matrix (ECM) deposition and degradation.

Within seconds, minutes, and hours after injury, epidermal and dermal cell migration, proliferation, and differentiation initiate re-epithelialization.[1] External injury may trigger tissue hypoxia, which leads to upregulation of local growth factors (cytokines), degradation of ECM, and may ultimately lead to angiogenesis. Newly formed granulation tissue must be sustained to establish the formation of new blood vessels.[2] Many diseases are related to keratinocyte or epidermal cell loss, angiogenesis dysfunction, and incomplete skin regeneration. These disorders including Buerger disease, chronic radiation wounds, and other chronic wound healing problems are under clinical investigation for possible new therapeutic modalities. Autologous adipose-derived stem cells (ADSCs) show great promise as an adjunct in facilitating the healing of these complex wounds.

Pathogenesis of Intractable or Nonhealing Wounds

Wound healing in skin comprises 4 major distinctive, but overlapping phases:

1. Hemostasis
2. Inflammatory
3. Proliferation
4. Remodeling.

Grant: Nagasaki University Global COE Program, "Global Strategic Center for Radiation Health Risk Control," by the Japan Society for the Promotion of Science.
[a] Department of Plastic and Reconstructive Surgery; [b] Takashi Nagai Memorial International Hibakusha Medical Center, Nagasaki University Hospital; [c] Department of Radiation Health Management, Fukushima Medical University, 1 Hikarigaoka, Fukushima, Japan; [d] Atomic Bomb Disease Institute, Nagasaki University School of Medicine
* Corresponding author. 1-7-1 Sakamoto, Nagasaki 852-8501, Japan.
E-mail address: akitas@hf.rim.or.jp

Clin Plastic Surg 39 (2012) 281–292
doi:10.1016/j.cps.2012.04.005

In a chronic wound, remarkable changes related to senescence, ischemia, matrix biology, and bacterial colonization transform the normal progression of wound healing into a self-continuing cycle of inflammation and injury.[3] Injured tissue induces tissue hypoxia, which leads to upregulation of growth factors; degradation of ECM activates local angiogenesis. Stem cells have shown to promote angiogenic processes.[4–6] Stem cells also may be differentiated into various cells including fibroblasts, which are major component of dermis.[7]

Chronic wounds include venous ulcers, pressure ulcers, and diabetic ulcers, which may account for 90% of all nonhealing wounds.[3]

Venous ulcers are highly prevalent in woman[8] and are related to circulatory insufficiency and venous hypertension located in and around the malleolus.

Pressure sores commonly occur in patients with impaired mobility and under prolonged medical and surgical care, such as extensive surgery, time spent in an intensive care unit, and poor systemic nutrition status. Pressure ulcers arise from external force, friction, and shear forces that affect segmental and perforator arteries leading to tissue necrosis particularly over bony prominences.[9]

Diabetic ulcers result in long-term complications in diabetic patients. Most ulcers in patients with diabetes are located in pressure points of the foot and can arise from peripheral neuropathy, foot deformity, and local minor trauma.[10] In a diabetic wound, ischemia can result from a macrovascular, microvascular, and neuropathic disease, or all the aforementioned.[11]

Chronic wounds are complicated and etiologically multifactorial. Ischemia-reperfusion injury may play a major and important role in etiology.[3] Ischemic stresses are altered in elderly people, partly because of the combination of ischemia and oxidant stresses in the ischemia-reperfusion injury.[12] Negative pressure wound therapy may prevent systemic damage caused by ischemic reperfusion, as demonstrated in a pig model.[13]

Wound healing contains multifactorial local and systemic factors. Wound bed preparation involves management of the following parameters[14]:

- Tissue viability
- Involvement of infection
- Moisture balance
- Wound edges.

In addition, local alteration of metalloproteinases, integrins, chemokines, and growth factors on the wound surface must be controlled.[15–17]

Treatment of Chronic Wounds

Treatment of chronic wounds is affected by optimal environmental conditions, the healing process, and subsequent scarring. Surgical or nonsurgical debridement, reduction of edema, diminishing bacterial burdens, maintaining the favorable moisture balance, and removal of undermining tissues are included in standard wound care.[18]

Wound characteristics can be modified with a variety of recently developed topical dressings such as impregnated gauze, film, hydrogel, hydrocolloid, and alginate. Advanced therapies include mechanical devices providing topical negative pressure and bioengineered tissues of various types.[19–23] Even though vigorous development of such materials, devices, and products are underway, surgical debridement is still required to facilitate wound healing. Debridement can reduce the bioburden of a wound selectively and effectively. Necrotic tissue, which must be eliminated because it behaves as a substrate for proliferating bacteria that strives for the same nutrients and oxygen molecules essential for wound healing, is best removed with debridement.

Stem Cells in Wound Healing

Stem cells are able to[24]

- Undergo self-renewal
- Be cell proliferative
- Differentiate into multiple lineages of cell and tissue phenotypes.

Recent technological developments now allow isolation and culture of stem cells, which has enabled researchers to perform vigorous studies on somatic or adult stem cells.

Adult stem cells can differentiate into adipogenic, osteogenic, and neurogenic cell types.[25] The autologous adult stem cells are readily available from the patient, thus not affected by ethical and immunologic barriers. Mesenchymal stem cells are first isolated from bone marrow and extend to almost all organs and tissues.[26,27] Bone marrow-derived stem cells (BMMSCs) from a single donor can differentiate into liver epithelium, lung, gastrointestinal tract, and skin.[28,29] BMMSCs are relatively easily obtained from bone-marrow aspirates of donor patients. BMMSCs are isolated and expanded in vitro by subculturing.[30] Human BMMSCs (hBMMSCs) are resistant to 20 Gy radiation in vitro; immediately after exposure to 20 Gy radiations and reconstruction with hBMMSCs and angiogenic growth factor (basic fibroblast growth factor, [bFGF]), artificial dermis demonstrated improved wound healing in 10 days.[31]

Case 1: Procedural radiation injury

A 58-year-old male patient had received 45 Gy of radiation and subsequently developed chest pain. He then underwent percutaneous transluminal coronary angioplasty under fluoroscopy, which was unexpectedly prolonged as a result of intraoperative complications. Immediately after the procedure, the patient noticed strong, deep, penetrating pain in his back. He subsequently developed a localized wound deep into the costal cartilage and a surrounding erythematic lesion, which was apparent at first follow-up surgical visit. The wound was widely excised including the necrotic cartilage and was reconstructed with a bilobed latissimus dorsi musculocutaneous flap. The scar tissue resulting from exposure to original radiation was further analyzed via histologic analysis. Small spindle-shaped cells were concentrated within the fibrotic tissue and Stro-1, which is one of the immunoreactive markers of mesenchymal stem cells.[32] This finding suggested that stem cells may mediate a radiation injury (**Fig. 1**).

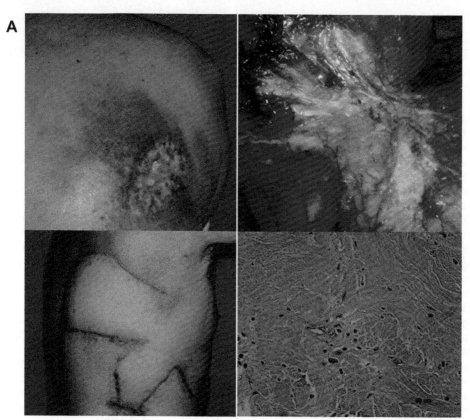

Fig. 1. STRO-1 immunoreactivity in the radiation-induced wound and subsequent scarring from a 58-year-old male patient's back. (*A*) (*upper left*) Radiation injury with exposed costal rib and central tissue necrosis at first visit, 2 years after fluoroscopic procedure. (*upper right*) In the reverse side of injury, scarring observed at periphery of the base was very hard. (*lower left*) 2 years after reconstruction by latissimus dorsi musculocutaneous flap (bilobed flap). (*lower right*) Small fusiform cells were abundant in the scar tissue. (*B*) Immunohistological analysis of STRO-1 in scarred tissue. In the right, scarred tissue explanting cell culture demonstrated STRO-1 immunoreactivity in cell cytoplasm.

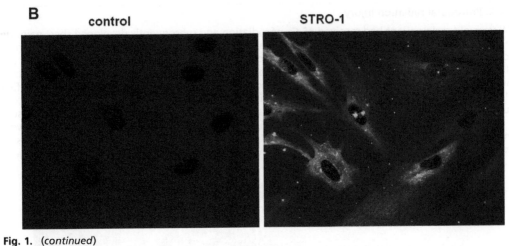

Fig. 1. (*continued*)

BMMSCs can synthesize higher amount of collagen, fibroblast growth factor (FGF), and vascular endothelial growth factor (VEGF), suggesting a potential benefit in accelerating wound healing.[33] hBMMSCs are able to accelerate wound healing with a collagen sponge with bFGF.[34] Over a 1-year observation of autologous bone marrow cell treatment for 3 nonhealing wounds, which previously failed to heal with the use of bioengineered skin or skin grafting, complete closure and dermal rebuilding in all cases was demonstrated with autologous bone marrow cell. Reduced scarring and engraftment of grafted cells was observed.[35] Fibrin polymer spray, in which fibrinogen contains cultured autologous BMMSCs, can adhere to the wound bed and retain the cell viability and migration.[36] Cultured BMMSCs are used for severe radiation-associated wounds with numerical dosimetry-guided surgery followed up to 11 months.[37] Also, cultured BMMSCs are effective for intractable wounds when soaked in an artificial dermis.[38] In addition, direct injection of cultured BMMSCs into the wound area in normal diabetic mice promoted wound healing through the release of proangiogenic factors on differentiation[39]; In streptozocin (STX)-induced diabetic rats, BMMSC double-system injections through the tail vein and local injection at the wound site augmented growth factors such as EGF, VEGF, platelet-derived growth factor-BB markedly and transforming growth factor-β and keratinocyte growth factor (KGF) moderately.[40,41] BMMSCs induce potent differentiation and proliferation under low oxygen tension with cell morphologic and cell cycle changes and differentiation capacity toward bone and fat.[42]

Furthermore, hBMMSCs transplantation to an adult rabbit incisional wound demonstrated tensile strength 80 days after surgery.[43] Systemic administration of rat BMMSCs for 4 days promotes wound healing, increases production of collagen, rapid maturation of wound, and increases the tensile strength.[44]

Stem cells are found in very low amounts among the nucleated cells from the bone marrow and even lesser amounts in the peripheral blood. Fibrocytes originate in bone marrow[45] and are found in peripheral blood, wounds, and tissue remodeling.[46] A recent study of peripheral blood demonstrated that fibrocytes are able to proliferate cells, and induce re-epithelialization and angiogenesis in a diabetic mouse.[17]

ADSCs

Fat tissues contain multipotent cells, with similar wound healing effects of BMMSCs, stimulating human dermal fibroblasts.[47] They have the capacity to differentiate into adipogenic, chondrogenic, myogenic, and osteogenic cell lineage when cultured in vitro with similar cell surface cluster of differentiation antigens.[48,49] ADSCs are obtained from either liposuction procedure or solid fat tissue. ADSCs are called adipose-derived regenerative cells because they contain heterogeneous inducible regenerative cells.[50] ADSCs are more easily obtained from the donor sites than BMMC and are extensively proliferative ex vivo in vitro. Fat tissue plays an important role in regulating energy balance and substance metabolism, and its biologic function in terms of metabolism, hormone, and signaling are varying.[51] In vitro, assay depending on the anatomic location of the donor sites, age, and gender may differ in yielding and differentiation capacity.[52] ADSCs are approximately 5000 CFU-F per gram of adipose tissue whereas the estimated CFU-F per milliliter of bone marrow is 100 to 1000.[53] Comparing lipoaspirate and excised adipose tissues, aspirated adipose tissue yields more preadipocytes within 60 minutes after extraction and at 24 hours storage at 4° than extracted tissue.[54] Although distinction of preadipocytes from ADSCs via lipoaspiration is still unknown, it is acknowledged that preadipocytes can be used for fat-based regeneration.[55] There are several reasons that ADSCs are most favorable cell sources for regeneration:

- The lipoaspiration procedure is relatively common for surgeons.
- ADSCs contain superior potentials to induce both angiogenesis and vasculogenesis.[56]
- In vivo studies prove the efficacy and effectiveness using ADSCs.[57]
- ADSCs are easily cultured and have high-affinity with three-dimensional scaffolds and other cells.[58]

ADSCs in Wound Healing

ADSCs are available for promoting angiogenesis, secreting growth factors and cytokines, and differentiating into multiple cell types on stimuli. ADSCs can promote human dermal fibroblast proliferation by directly contacting cells and paracrine activation in re-epithelialization phase of wound healing.[47] Two-dimensional gel electrophoretic gel proteomic analysis of the intracellular protein of BMMSCs and ADSCs revealed that the proteins were similar, which suggests that ADSCs can replace BMMSCs in cell therapy.[59] In mice, wounds healed faster when treated with ADSCs than with normal process. In nonirradiated and locally irradiated wounds in mouse, ADSCs can be differentiated to keratinocytes and produce KGF as well as vascular endothelial growth factor (VEGF).[60] ADSCs can release angiogenic factors in ischemic injury. ADSCs in acellular dermal matrix provide a framework for support of the regenerative capacity in wound healing.[61] With appropriate scaffolds, ADSCs can cause regeneration and induce wound healing. ADSCs with skin substitute containing human ECM can produce subcutaneous, dermal, and epidermal regenerated tissues.[62] Using clinically available human acellular dermal matrix of cadaveric donors, ADSCs demonstrated accelerated wound healing by 7 days postoperatively and microvascular endothelial phenotype for 2 weeks, indicating the direct vascular networking in tissue regeneration with no systemic distribution other than surgical engrafted sites.[63]

In a diabetic mouse model, noncultured excised ADSCs with commercially available bilayer artificial dermis can secrete several growth factors and cytokines for 4 days in cell culture supernatants, and histologic examination demonstrated advanced granulation tissue formation, capillary formation, and epithelialization for 2 weeks postoperatively.[64]

In a pig multiple full-thickness wound model, cultured ADSCs with platelet-rich plasma can enhance the wound healing process in terms of VEGF concentration in the fluid and cosmetic appearance.[65] ADSCs are able to demonstrate antioxidant effect via dermal fibroblasts and keratinocytes in a paracrine manner,[66] and hypoxia increases VEGF and bFGF levels as well as induces cell proliferation.[67]

ADIPOSE-DERIVED REGENERATIVE CELL THERAPY FOR CHRONIC RADIATION INJURY
Background of Adipose-Derived Regenerative Cell Therapy

Although literature emphasizes the merit and advantage of the use of ADSCs or adipose-derived regenerative cells (ADRCs) in wound healing, at present, there are few clinical applications. Autologous cultured BMMSCs are now being used to treat severe radiation injury.[68] The purified autologous lipoaspirates are injected to improve radiation ulcers.[69]

Nagasaki University Global Strategic Center for Radiation Health Risk Control

This clinical study project is designed under Nagasaki University Global Strategic Center for Radiation Health Risk Control, which is one of the global center-of-excellence programs funded by the Ministry of Education, Culture, Sports and Technology from 2007 to 2011. The aim of this program is to focus on global assessment of radiation and effect to health risk, to overcome the legacy of atomic bombing, to establish the scientific basis of human safety to radiation, and to promote international collaboration that will nurture the experts in this field. To accomplish these aims 3 research projects are set:

1. Radiation and nuclear basic life science research
2. Atomic bomb disease medical research
3. International radiation health science research.

The goal of this project was to establish the scientific basis of radiation health risk control to contribute to society through Hibaku/Hibakusha (radiation-exposed) medicine. Radiation based life science research investigates external and internal irradiation, mechanisms of chronic low-dose radiation, risk assessment and management, susceptibility, and racial difference in individual risk assessment. Atomic bomb disease medical research deals with aging of the atomic bomb survivors who have progressive cancer, multiple cancer, and psychosomatic effects and also treating foreign Hibakusha atomic bomb survivors. International radiation health science research handles broad aspects of threat of nuclear events, global nuclear power plant (NPP) accidents and disasters, and world health organization-radiation emergency medical assistance and networking (WHO-REMPAN) collaboration center activity. Through WHO-REMPAN collaboration center, development and clinical application of regenerative medicine is further promoted (**Fig. 2**). Because

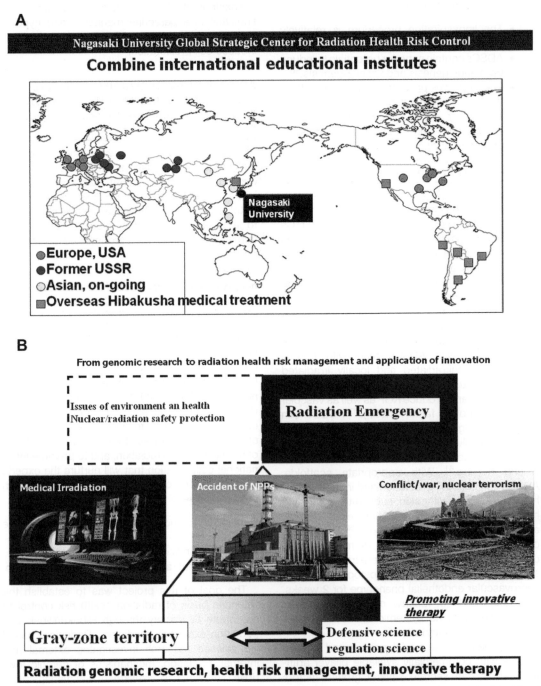

Fig. 2. Scheme of Nagasaki University Global Strategic Center for Radiation Health Risk Control. (*A*) Global focal points of collaboration with Nagasaki University. (*B*) Strategy applying to promoting innovative therapy such as ADSCs for radiation injury is a part of this project.

acute systemic radiation injuries are rare and unpredictable, the possibility of applying patients' own fat tissue–derived stem cell therapy of their subcutaneous tissues not exposed to radiation for chronic local radiation injury is attempted.

Patient Enrollment

Five clinical treatment experiences with autologous noncultured ADSCs for more than 18 months, which is considered the final phase of wound healing remodeling process,[1] mean patients' follow-up period was 2 years ± 6 months (2 years 10 months to 1 year 9 months) postoperatively. All 5 patients, who were women, healed uneventfully, average healing 8 ± 2.2 weeks, among which 1 patient

was treated for her consistent pain in her left toes as a result of thromboangiitis due to Buerger disease. Mean age of the patients were 64.4 ± 22.0. There is no recurrence or abnormal wound healing during follow-up periods in any of the patients.

Surgical Procedure, Scaffold (Artificial Dermis), and Growth Factor

In adipose-derived stem cell transplantation and postoperative management, an artificial dermis (Terudermis, Olympus-Terumo Biomaterials Corp, Ltd, Japan) was used as a scaffold. Terudermis comprises 2 layers: a lower layer of bovine atelocollagen and an upper layer comprising a silicone

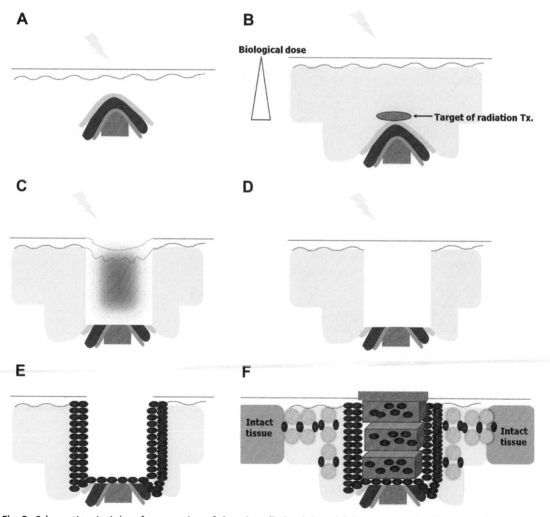

Fig. 3. Schematic principles of progression of chronic radiation injury. (*A*) Once external radiation is administered. (*B*) For therapeutic radiation, dose is usually greater for target organs located deeper in the tissue. (*C*) Radiated tissue is getting sclerotic in process of chronic radiation injury. (*D*) Surgical debridement is aimed at the wounded and most severe areas. (*E*) ADSCs are injected or soaked around wound margins and wound bed. (*F*) Stacked artificial dermis (Terudermis) and liposuctioned adipose tissue mixed with ADSCs are bridged with the adjacent intact tissue.

Case 2: Radiation injury resulting from cancer treatment

An 87-year-old woman was treated for uterine cervical cancer. 50 Gy of two-gate radiation was performed 40 years previously. The wound reached to the sacral bone, paravertebral muscles and ligaments. The radiation injury caused central wounding and massive exudation. Several surgical treatments were performed with artificial dermis alone, artificial dermis with bFGF or split-thickness skin grafting. None was successful and wounding recurred within several weeks. The most severe part of wound was surgically debrided and 3.7×10^7 cells were injected at the edges and the base. The fat tissue mixed cells bridged between the wound margin and intact tissue. The wound was covered with Terudermis and the outer membrane remained in place for 1 week, then bFGF was sprayed. The wound healed 72 days post-operatively. Hypertrophic scar developed at 180 days, but there is no hypertrophic scar or recurrence of wound at 970 days postoperatively. A small portion of the processed cells is cultured in vitro for confirmation of cell proliferation and capacity of differentiation. The cultured cells demonstrated stem cell properties (**Figs. 4** and **5**).

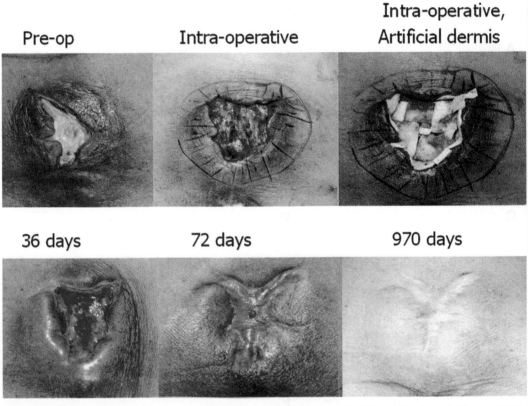

Fig. 4. An 87-year-old woman was treated for uterine cervical cancer. A 50 Gy of 2 gate radiation was performed 40 years ago and wound was reached to the sacral bone, muscle, and ligament: (*A*) Preoperative, (*B*) Intraoperative, (*C*) Intraoperative with artificial dermis, (*D*) 36 days, (*E*) 72 days with linear hypertrophic scar formation, and (*F*) 970 days wound healed and pliable.

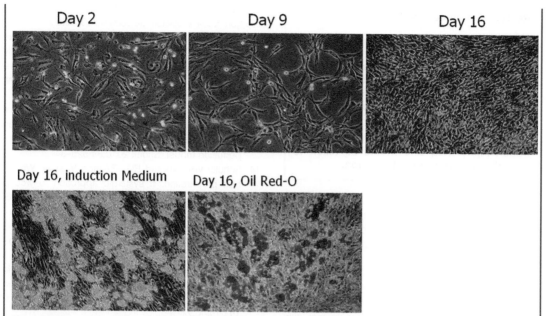

Fig. 5. In vitro cell proliferation and differentiation. (*Upper left*) Adipose-derived stem cells in regular cell culture medium at day 2. (*Upper center*) Adipose-derived stem cells in ES cell culture medium at day 9. (*Upper right*) Adipose-derived stem cells in ES cell culture medium at day 16 at confluent. (*Lower left*) Adipose-derived stem cells in ES cell culture medium at day 16 by differentiation induction. (*Lower right*) Adipose-derived stem cells in ES cell culture medium at day 16, lipid is marled in red by Oil-Red O staining (original magnification ×100).

sheet, which protects against infection and dryness from the outside.

- After minimum debridement, Terudermis was multilayered and stacked over freshly debrided wounds.
- The silicone sheets were removed except top Terudermis.
- Two-thirds of isolated ADSCs were injected around the debrided wound at the base of the wounds, and into Terudermis.
- Another one-third of ADSCs was mixed with the autologous adipose tissue, which was rinsed with a lactated Ringer solution.
- In the Celution system, after isolating ADSCs, the disposable cell collection plastic case was again used to mix the suctioned fat, which is rinsed separately in the 50-cc syringe and repeated until the oil droplets are removed.
- After being mixed, it was injected into a zone of hard fibrotic tissue around the debrided wounds in 2-cm width in all directions.

Pearls and pitfalls regarding stem cell treatment

ADSCs are relatively easy to harvest and process.

In very lean patients, ADSCs may need to be cultured.

Detailed surgical procedure is described in the literature.[70] Briefly, surgical debridement is limited to the most severely affected area in depth and in width. The cells are injected at the edges and the base, evenly washed fat tissue mixed with cells are injected to bridge between the wound and intact tissue (**Fig. 3**).

Angiogenic growth factor, bFGF, and genetically recombinant human bFGF (Fiblast, Trafermin) were purchased from Kaken Pharmaceutical Co., Inc (Tokyo, Japan). The freeze-dried bFGF was dissolved in 5 mL of benzalkonium chloride–containing solution right before the first use and stored at 4°C for 1 day, with 300 μL sprayed over an area of 30 cm^2 from 5 cm distance and 0.3 mL/d of this solution was applied over the wound when the outer layer of the artificial dermis is naturally peeled off and administration of bFGF starts 3 to

---

First-person experience with stem cell treatment by author

- Active ADSCs can be harvested in elderly patients.
- In cell culture, these cells are able to proliferate and differentiate into adipose tissue.
- Even an 87-year-old patient was able to heal a radiation-related ulcer of the sacrum with the assistance of ADSCs.

> **Stem cell techniques pearls**
>
> - The harvesting equipment is configured in a closed circuit to minimize the risk of contamination. When harvesting subcutaneous adipose tissue, one should be cautious to not penetrate into deeper structures such as visceral cavity in abdomen or major muscles, vessels, and nerves.
> - While injecting ADSCs/ADRCs in chronic radiation injury sites, care should be taken to avoid surface rupture or laceration.

7 days postoperatively. The wound was covered with nonadherent occlusive foam dressing.

All cases demonstrated complete wound healing by 10 weeks postoperatively.

REFERENCES

1. Martin P. Wound healing-aiming for perfect skin regeneration. Science 1997;276:75–81.
2. Brem H, Tomic-Canic M. Cellular and molecular basis of wound healing in diabetes. J Clin Invest 2007;117: 1219–22.
3. Mustoe T, O'Shaughnessy K, Kloeters O. Chronic wound pathogenesis and current treatment strategies: a unifying hypothesis. Plast Reconstr Surg 2006;117(Suppl 7):S35–41.
4. Hanjaya-Putra D, Gerecht S. Vascular engineering using human embryonic stem cells. Biotechnol Prog 2009;25:2–9.
5. Sorrell J, Baber M, Caplan A. Influence of adult mesenchymal stem cells on in vitro vascular formation. Tissue Eng Part A 2009;15:1751–61.
6. Wu Q, Shao H, Darwin ED, et al. Extracellular calcium increases CXCR4 expression on bone marrow-derived cells and enhances pro-angiogenesis therapy. J Cell Mol Med 2009;13:3764–73.
7. Watkins S, Zippin J. When wound healing goes awry. A review of normal and abnormal wound healing, scar pathophysiology and therapeutics. J Drugs Dermatol 2008;7:997–1005.
8. Heit J, Rooke T, Silverstein M, et al. Trends in the incidence of venous stasis syndrome and venous ulcer: a 25-year population-based study. J Vasc Surg 2001;33:1022–7.
9. Rogers A, Burnett S, Moore J, et al. Involvement of proteolytic enzymes–plasminogen activators and matrix metalloproteinases–in the pathophysiology of pressure ulcers. Wound Repair Regen 1995;3: 273–83.
10. Boulton AJ. The diabetic foot: a global view. Diabetes Metab Res Rev 2000;16(Suppl 1):S2–5.
11. Gershater MA, Londahl M, Nyberg P, et al. Complexity of factors related to outcome of neuropathic and neuroischaemic/ischaemic diabetic foot ulcers: a cohort study. Diabetologia 2009;52:398–407.
12. Mogford JE, Liu WR, Reid R, et al. Adenoviral human telomerase reverse transcriptase dramatically improves ischemic wound healing without detrimental immune response in an aged rabbit model. Hum Gene Ther 2006;17:651–60.
13. Kubiak BD, Albert SP, Gatto AL, et al. Peritoneal negative pressure therapy prevents multiple organ injury in a chronic porcine sepsis and ischemia/reperfusion model. Shock 2010;34:525–34.
14. Schultz GS, Sibbald RG, Falanga V, et al. Wound bed preparation: a systemic approach to wound management. Wound Repair Regen 2003;11:S1–28.
15. Nedeau AE, Gallagher KA, Liu ZJ, et al. Elevation of hemopexin-like fragment of matrix metalloproteinase-2 tissue levels inhibits ischemic wound healing and angiogenesis. J Vasc Surg 2011;54:1430–8.
16. Hamed S, Ulmann Y, Egozi D, et al. Fibronectin potentiates topical erythropoietin-induced wound repair in diabetic mice. J Invest Dermatol 2011; 131:1365–74.
17. Kao HK, Chen B, Murphy GF, et al. Peripheral blood fibrocytes: enhancement of wound healing by cell proliferation, re-epithelialization, contraction, and angiogenesis. Ann Surg 2011;254:1066–74.
18. Ligresiti C, Bo F. Wound bed preparation of difficult wounds: an evolution of the principles of TIME. Int Wound J 2007;4:21–9.
19. Macri L, Clark RA. Tissue engineering for cutaneous wounds: selecting the proper time and space for growth factors, cells and the extracellular matrix. Skin Pharmacol Physiol 2009;22:83–93.
20. Smiell JM, Wieman TJ, Steed DL, et al. Efficacy and safety of becaplermin (recombinant human platelet-derived growth factor-BB) in patients with nonhealing, lower extremity diabetic ulcers: a combined analysis of four randomized studies. Wound Repair Regen 1998;7:335–46.
21. Robson MC, Phillips LG, Lawrence WT, et al. The safety and effect of topically applied recombinant basic fibroblast growth factor on healing of chronic pressure sores. Ann Surg 1992;216:401–16.
22. Marston WA, Hanft J, Norwood P, et al. The efficacy and safety of Dermagraft in improving the healing of chronic diabetic foot ulcers: results of a prospective randomized trial. Diabetes Care 2003;26:1701–5.
23. Falanga V, Sabolinksi M. A bilayered living skin construct (APLIGRAF) accelerates complete closure of hard-to-heal venous ulcers. Wound Repair Regen 1999;7:201–7.
24. Anderson DJ, Gage FH, Weissman IL. Can stem cells cross lineage boundaries? Nat Med 2001;7:393–5.
25. Montanucci P, Basta G, Pescara T, et al. New simple and rapid method for purification of mesenchymal stem cells from the human umbilical cord Wharton jelly. Tissue Eng Part A 2011;17:2651–61.

26. Pittenger MF, McKay SC, Beck RK, et al. Multilineage potential of adult human mesenchymal stem cells. Science 1999;284:143–7.

27. da Silva Meirelles L, Chagastelles PC, Nardi NB. Mesenchymal stem cells reside in virtually all postnatal organs and tissues. J Cell Sci 2006;119(Pt 11):2204–13.

28. Krause DS, Theise ND, Collector MI, et al. Multiorgan, multilineage engraftment by a single bone marrow-derived stem cell. Cell 2001;105:369–77.

29. Badiavas EV, Abedi M, Butmarc J, et al. Participation of bone marrow derived cells in cutaneous wound healing. J Cell Physiol 2003;196:245–50.

30. Barry FP, Murphy JM. Mesenchymal stem cells: clinical applications and biological characterization. Int J Cell Biol 2004;36:568–84.

31. Akita S, Akino K, Hirano A, et al. Mesenchymal stem cell therapy for cutaneous radiation syndrome. Health Phys 2010;98:858–62.

32. Ning H, Lin G, Lue TF, et al. Mesenchymal stem cell marker Stro-1 is a 75kd endothelial antigen. Biochem Biophys Res Commun 2011;413:353–7.

33. Han SK, Yoon TH, Lee DG, et al. Potential of human bone marrow stromal cells to accelerate wound healing in vitro. Ann Plast Surg 2005;55:414–9.

34. Nakagawa H, Akita S, Fukui M, et al. Human mesenchymal stem cells successfully improve skin-substitute wound healing. Br J Dermatol 2005;153:29–36.

35. Badiavas EV, Falanga V. Treatment of chronic wounds with bone marrow-derived cells. Arch Dermatol 2003;139:510–6.

36. Falanga V, Iwamoto S, Chartier M, et al. Autologous bone marrow-derived cultured mesenchymal stem cells delivered in a fibrin spray accelerates healing in murine and human cutaneous wounds. Tissue Eng 2007;13:1299–312.

37. Lataillade JJ, Doucet C, Bey E, et al. New approach to radiation burn treatment by dosimetry-guided surgery combined with autologous mesenchymal stem cell therapy. Regen Med 2007;2:785–94.

38. Yoshikawa T, Mitsuno H, Nonaka I, et al. Wound therapy by marrow mesenchymal cell transplantation. Plast Reconstr Surg 2008;121:860–77.

39. Wu Y, Chen L, Scott PG, et al. Mesenchymal stem cells enhance wound healing through differentiation and angiogenesis. Stem Cells 2007;25:2648–59.

40. Kwon DS, Gao X, Liu YB, et al. Treatment with bone marrow-derived stromal cells accelerates wound healing in diabetic rats. Int Wound J 2008;5:453–63.

41. Sasaki M, Abe R, Fujita Y, et al. Mesenchymal stem cells are recruited into wounded skin and contribute to wound repair by transdifferentiation into multiple skin cell type. J Immunol 2008;180:2581–7.

42. Ren H, Cao Y, Zhao Q, et al. Proliferation and differentiation of bone marrow stromal cells under hypoxic conditions. Biochem Biophys Res Commun 2006;347:12–21.

43. Stoff A, Rivera AA, Sanjib Banerjee N, et al. Promotion of incisional wound repair by human mesenchymal stem cell transplantation. Exp Dermatol 2009;18:362–9.

44. McFarlin K, Gao X, Liu YB, et al. Bone marrow-derived mesenchymal stromal cells accelerates wound healing in the rat. Wound Repair Regen 2006;14:471–8.

45. Mori L, Bellini A, Stacey MA, et al. Fibrocytes contribute to the myofibroblast population in wounded skin and originate from the bone marrow. Exp Cell Res 2005;304:81–90.

46. Bucala R, Spiegel LA, Chesney J, et al. Circulating fibrocytes define a new leukocyte subpopulation that mediates tissue repair. Mol Med 1994;1:71–81.

47. Kim WS, Park BS, Sung JH, et al. Wound healing effect of adipose-derived stem cells: a critical role of secretory factors on human dermal fibroblasts. J Dermatol Sci 2007;48:15–24.

48. Zuk PA, Zhu M, Mizuno H, et al. Multilineage cells from human adipose tissue: implications for cell-based therapies. Tissue Eng 2001;7:21–8.

49. Zuk PA, Zhu M, Ashjian P, et al. Human adipose tissue is a source of multipotent stem cells. Mol Biol Cell 2002;13:4279–95.

50. Kondo K, Shintani S, Shibata R, et al. Implantation of adipose-derived regenerative cells enhances ischemia-induced angiogenesis. Arterioscler Thromb Vasc Biol 2009;29:61–6.

51. Giorgino F, Laviola L, Eriksson JW. Regional differences of insulin action in adipose tissue: insights from in vivo and in vitro studies. Acta Physiol Scand 2005;183:13–30.

52. Schipper BM, Marra KG, Zhang W, et al. Regional anatomic and age effects on cell function of human adipose-derived stem cells. Ann Plast Surg 2008;60:538–44.

53. Strem BM, Hicok KC, Zhu M, et al. Multipotential differentiation of adipose tissue-derived stem cells. Keio J Med 2005;54:132–41.

54. von Heimburgh D, Hemmrich K, Haydarlioglu S, et al. Comparison of viable cell yield form excised versus aspirated adipose tissue. Cells Tissues Organs 2004;178:87–92.

55. Tholpady SS, Aojanepong C, Llull R, et al. The cellular plasticity of human adipocytes. Ann Plast Surg 2005;54:651–6.

56. Nie C, Yang D, Xu J, et al. Locally administered adipose-derived stem cells accelerate wound healing through differentiation and vasculogenesis. Cell Transplant 2011;20:205–16.

57. Strem BM, Hedrick MH. The growing importance of fat in regenerative medicine. Trends Biotechnol 2005;23:64–6.

58. Neofytou EA, Chang E, Patlola B, et al. Adipose tissue-derived stem cells display a proangiogenic

phenotype on 3D scaffolds. J Biomed Mater Res A 2011;98:383–93.

59. Roche S, Delorme B, Oostendorp RA, et al. Comparative proteomic analysis of human mesenchymal and embryonic stem cells: towards the definition of a mesenchymal stem cell proteomic structure. Proteomics 2009;9:232–3.

60. Ebrahimian TG, Pouzoulet F, Squiban C, et al. Cell theory based on adipose tissue-derived stromal cells promotes physiological and pathological wound healing. Arterioscler Thromb Vasc Biol 2009;29:503–10.

61. Nie C, Yang D, Morris SF. Local delivery of adipose-derived stem cells via acellular dermal matrix as a scaffold: a new promising strategy to accelerate wound healing. Med Hypotheses 2009;72:679–82.

62. Trottier V, Marceau-Fortier G, Germain L, et al. IFATS collection: Using human adipose-derived stem/stromal cells for the production of new skin substitutes. Stem Cells 2008;26:2713–23.

63. Altman AM, Matthias N, Yan Y, et al. Dermal matrix as a carrier for in vivo delivery of human adipose-derived stem cells. Biomaterials 2008;29:1431–42.

64. Nambu M, Kishimoto S, Muzuno H, et al. Accelerated wound healing in healing-impaired db/db mice by autologous adipose tissue-derived stromal cells combined with atelocollagen matrix. Ann Plast Surg 2009;62:317–21.

65. Blanton M, Hadad I, Johnstone B, et al. Adipose stromal cells and platelet-rich plasma therapies synergistically increase revascularization during wound healing. Plast Reconsr Surg 2009;123(Suppl 2):56S–64S.

66. Kim WS, Park BS, Sung JH. The wound-healing and antioxidant effects of adipose-derived stem cells. Expert Opin Biol Tjer 2009;9:879–87.

67. Lee EY, Xia Y, Kim WS, et al. Hypoxia-enhanced wound-healing function of adipose-derived stem cells: increase in stem cell proliferation and upregulation of VEGF and bFGF. Wound Repair Regen 2009;17:540–7.

68. Bey E, Prat M, Duhamel P, et al. Emerging therapy for improving wound repair of severe radiation burns using local bone marrow-derived stem cell administrations. Wound Repair Regen 2010;18:50–8.

69. Rigotti G, Marchi A, Galie M, et al. Clinical treatment of radiotherapy tissue damage by lipoaspirate transplant: a healing process mediated by adipose-derived adult stem cells. Plast Reconostr Surg 2007;119:1409–22.

70. Akita S, Akino K, Hirano A, et al. Noncultured autologous adipose-derived stem cells therapy for chronic radiation injury. Stem Cells Int 2010;2010:52704.

Oxygen in Wound Healing
Nutrient, Antibiotic, Signaling Molecule, and Therapeutic Agent

David E. Eisenbud, MD

KEYWORDS

- Oxygen • Hypoxia • Hyperbaric • Wound • Healing • Diabetes • Epithelium • Fibroblast

KEY POINTS

- With deeper scientific understanding of oxygen physiology, and with support from randomized, prospective clinical investigations, the judicious, individualized use of oxygen therapy in wound management may now be considered mainstream.
- Each of the most common categories of chronic wounds (arterial, venous, diabetic, pressure) become established or are perpetuated because of factors that limit oxygen delivery to the wound bed.
- At the low physiologic concentration of H_2O_2 (0.15%), topical angiogenesis is favorably influenced, distinguished from the 3% v/v strength available commercially; at this high concentration, severe oxidative damage to wounds is noted, and is thus contraindicated in modern wound management.
- Given that correction of wound hypoxia is beneficial to many aspects of healing, it does not necessarily follow that more is better, and that hyperoxygenation of normally nourished wounds confers a benefit to justify the risks.

INTRODUCTION

Common observations made many decades ago by mountain climbers who noted the inability to clear skin infections at high altitude, and Jacques Cousteau's deep sea divers who noted that their work wounds healed fastest when they were diving, brought general appreciation of the importance of oxygen in healing.[1] Recent years have brought an increased and more detailed scientific appreciation of the diverse roles that oxygen plays in normal physiology and disease states.[2,3] As the individual steps of the wound healing cascade have become elucidated in greater detail, the involvement of oxygen at nearly every stage has become evident. More oxygen is not always better; nature seems to have adapted us to respond constructively to the relative hypoxia that characterizes the healing edge of many wounds.

There remain many gaps in understanding of the biochemical events of healing. Some of the current knowledge regarding oxygen, growth factors, and other mediators is seemingly contradictory, and classification of molecules as promoters or inhibitors of healing (eg, oxygen is good, tumor necrosis factor α [TNF-α] is bad) is simplistic. However, it seems possible to reach a unified understanding of healing that reconciles most of the thousands of basic science investigations into individual steps in the chain, and oxygen is central to this. This article summarizes oxygen physiology in wound biology, and discusses the supporting literature.

Given the central role of oxygen in healing, there is the potential to manipulate the wound

The author has no financial conflicts of interest to declare in relation to the writing and publication of this article.
Millburn Surgical Associates, 225 Millburn Avenue, Suite 104-B, Millburn, NJ 07041, USA
E-mail address: dave@njdave.net

environment by treatment with supplemental oxygen. Oxygen therapy in various forms has been used to ameliorate many medical conditions for centuries. However, clinical results have been varied, and frequently disappointing. There has been an indiscriminate use of oxygen treatments in the past, and there is still an aura of quackery associated with this area of medicine. However, in the face of deeper scientific understanding of oxygen physiology, and with support from randomized, prospective clinical investigations, the judicious, individualized use of oxygen therapy in wound management may now be considered mainstream. This article reviews the current rationale, regimens, and preclinical and patient data regarding various oxygen treatments that have been used to improve the outcomes of dermal wounds. See **Box 1** for a summary of roles of oxygen in wound healing.

Oxygen Delivery

In normal conditions, oxygen delivery to peripheral tissues is the net result of:

- Cardiac output
- Peripheral vascular resistance
- Oxygen saturation of hemoglobin (usually 90% or greater).

Oxygen in serum
Minimal amounts of oxygen are dissolved in the serum. Release of oxygen is governed by the hemoglobin dissociation curve. Serum Po_2 is typically about 100 mm Hg. Once released at the

---

Box 1
Roles of oxygen in healing

- Energy source to fuel biochemical reactions and cellular function

- Nutrient essential to the synthesis and cross-linking of collagen

- Cofactor that is manufactured into signaling molecules such as nitric oxide and hydrogen peroxide

- Substrate for generation of reactive oxygen species (ROS) that combat wound colonization and infection

- Essential component of the redox switch that turns on and off genes that encode proteins critical to the healing cascade

- Deliberate hyperoxygenation recruits endothelial progenitor cells to the wound, increases vascular endothelial growth factor (VEGF), and promotes angiogenesis

---

capillary level into normal tissue, oxygen can diffuse up to 64 μm.[4] Given normal capillary density, this diffusion ability is sufficient to nourish and support the viability of the skin. Hunt[1] emphasized the often-neglected but relevant point that oxygen delivery can sometimes be increased significantly by reversing the local vasoconstriction that may result from pain, cold, or other noxious stimuli.

Intact skin as barrier to oxygen
The keratin layer of intact epithelium is a barrier to oxygen diffusion; probes designed to exclude air detect only 0 to 10 mm Hg on the skin surface. Warming of the skin makes this layer more permeable and enables Po_2 to increase substantially, although it does not reach the ambient level. Stripping the statum corneum with tape enables free diffusion of oxygen into the upper layers of dermis, and the Po_2 there closely matches the oxygen tension in the environment. However, within about a day, exudation of serum and accumulation of inflammatory cells lead to formation of a soft eschar that again prevents oxygen diffusion into the skin. Therefore, the oxygen tension in subcutaneous tissue and dermis of intact skin depends on delivery through the underlying circulatory system.

Inadequate Oxygen Delivery is a Causal Factor in Many Chronic Wounds

Each of the most common categories of chronic wounds (arterial, venous, diabetic, pressure) become established or are perpetuated because of factors that limit oxygen delivery to the wound bed. Scheffield[5] noted that chronic wounds have a Po_2 in the range of 5 to 20 mm Hg, compared with 35 to 50 mm Hg measured in normal tissue.

In the case of venous leg ulceration, the essential disturbance is abnormal venous hypertension, which is propagated back to the capillary level. The capillary-tissue pressure gradient is increased, causing water to diffuse out of the intravascular space and into the interstitium; large molecules such as fibrinogen, albumin, and α2-macroglobulin are also forced out of the vascular system, and pericapillary cuffs are formed that can be noted histologically.[6] These cuffs and the local edema impair oxygen diffusion and render the cells furthest from the capillary hypoxic.

Lower extremity arterial and diabetic wounds, are prone to suffer macrovascular and/or microvascular occlusive disease, limiting blood flow and therefore oxygen delivery to the lesion. Pressure wounds that are not properly off-loaded become ischemic (and therefore also hypoxic) when capillary closing pressure is exceeded by the weight of the body part pressing against a support surface.

Reperfusion

In addition to ischemia/hypoxia, another mechanism of injury has been shown to play a major role in a variety of chronic wounds: reperfusion.[6,7] Patients with impaired arterial inflow or venous return have repeated episodes of ischemia and reperfusion related to leg elevation or dependency. Restoring circulation induces endothelial stickiness, which draws white cells into the lesion; the already established proinflammatory environment established by ischemia intensifies as ROS flood the wound and cause further tissue destruction. Repeated episodes of ischemia and reperfusion are more detrimental to wound healing than are prolonged phases of uninterrupted ischemia.[8,9]

Inflammatory cycle

It is a popular current concept that many chronic wounds are stuck in a self-perpetuating inflammatory cycle. Hypoxia may contribute to this pathophysiology in many cases. Under significant hypoxic conditions, mitochondrial adenosine-triphosphate (ATP) production ceases and ATP-dependent transmembrane transport systems such as sodium/potassium ATPase or calcium ATPase fail. Intracellular accumulation of calcium promotes release of proinflammatory cytokines such as TNF-α and interleukin (IL)-1, which attract neutrophils and macrophages. Endothelial adhesion molecules are overexpressed in hypoxia, and enable white blood cells to localize to the wound. The net effect is a self-perpetuating inflammatory vicious cycle in which tissue destruction leads to increased white cell recruitment and release of proinflammatory mediators and ROS, which leads to even more tissue destruction.[7] Bacterial colonization, a nearly universal feature of chronic wounds, adds to the inflammatory burden by attracting and activating leukocytes. Although inflammatory cells are capable of producing ROS at low oxygen tensions, the antidotes to ROS (the most potent of which is nitric oxide) require higher oxygen tension for their synthesis.

Measurement of Wound Oxygen

Accurate, repeatable measurements of wound oxygen are central to many in vivo investigations into the role of oxygen. Although numerous investigators have refined research-grade systems, measurement of oxygen at the tissue/cellular level in routine clinical practice is difficult and imprecise. There is a vast literature on oxygen measurement and a detailed review is beyond the scope of this article. Most methods are indirect and measure oxygenation of periwound skin rather than the wound bed.

Transcutaneous oximetry

Perhaps the most popular of these techniques, transcutaneous oximetry ($TcPo_2$) is subject to high variability related to fluctuations in vasomotor tone at the site of measurement, light penetration of skin, and hemoglobin level.[7] Even perfectly performed $TcPo_2$ typically overestimates wound Po_2 because the skin is warmed to the point of maximal local vasodilatation, which is not representative of the ordinary state of the local vasculature. In addition, there can be significant oxygen consumption along the path from periwound intact skin to the healing tissue edge in the center of the wound.[10] Thus, arterial blood Po_2 is ordinarily about 100 mm Hg; the Po_2 of dermal wounds ranges from 60 mm Hg at the periphery to 0 to 10 mm Hg centrally. There are many reports supporting the usefulness of $TcPo_2$ in determining levels of amputation healing, but many practitioners have found that the method is cumbersome and yields results that have poor repeatability.[3,11] Measurements at 1 point in time and only a limited number of skin sites may not accurately portray the wound microenvironment, because wounds are not uniform and vasomotor tone may change from moment to moment.[12]

Luminescence imaging

Luminescence lifetime imaging has recently shown significant advantages compared with earlier methods of wound oxygen estimation.[7] A phosphorescent indicator is held in place on a plastic matrix; quenching of the phosphorescence is proportional to the amount of oxygen present. The technology provides a noninvasive, painless, reliable, sensitive estimate of wound Po_2.[13] Although offering potential for widespread clinical adoption, the technology is not yet available commercially in a format and at a cost that is compatible with ordinary clinic operations and economics.

Role of Oxygen in the Essential Steps of Dermal Wound Healing

Collagen synthesis

Extracellular matrix deposition is inadequate in many chronic wounds because of poor fibroblast production and inadequate remodeling of collagen, which are both oxygen dependent, and because of excessive degradation of extracorporeal membrane oxygenation (ECM) by matrix metalloproteinases (MMPs). Molecular oxygen is required for the hydroxylation of proline and lysine during collagen synthesis and for the maturation of protocollagen into stable triple-helical collagen. In the absence of sufficient oxygen, only protocollagen, which does not have the functional abilities of collagen, can be made.[2] Collagen synthesis proceeds in direct relation to Po_2 over the range of 25 to 250 mm Hg.[10,12] Prolyl hydroxylase under 20 mm Hg O_2 functions at 20% of maximal speed; the enzyme requires more than 150 mm Hg to reach 90% of maximal speed.[4,14]

Angiogenesis

Many authorities have noted an apparent inconsistency in well-known observations of wound healing, whereby hypoxia is noted to increase VEGF production from fibroblasts and macrophages, but angiogenesis seems to proceed more successfully under normoxic or even hyperoxic conditions.[12,15,16] In one set of instructive experiments, mice underwent subcutaneous injection of a gel alone, gel with VEGF, or with anti-VEGF antibodies. The animals were then maintained in various environments of 13% to 100% oxygen at 1 absolute atmosphere (ATA) to 2.8 ATA to simulate hypoxia, normoxia, and hyperoxia. The explanted gel plugs were then sectioned and graded for the degree of angiogenesis. Angiogenesis was significantly decreased in the hypoxic animals ($P = .001$) and increased in those who were rendered hyperoxic ($P<.05$). Addition of VEGF to the implanted gel did not prevent the deleterious effect of hypoxia. In contrast, the beneficial effect of hyperoxia was blocked by anti-VEGF antibody. These findings suggest that both adequate oxygen and the presence of VEGF are required for angiogenesis.

Sen[12] noted that all developing vascular buds require a sheath of ECM, mainly consisting of collagen and proteoglycans, to guide tube formation and resist the pressures of blood flow. His investigations have confirmed that optimal angiogenesis requires high Po_2; hypoxia, by retarding synthesis of the collagen to support developing vessels, decreases angiogenesis.[12]

Fibroblast growth

Oxygen consumption by cells has been studied by measuring changes in oxygen tension in supernatant media covering cells in tissue culture.[4] Fibroblast cellular proliferation is directly correlated with ambient oxygen level:

- Freshly harvested cells only grow in an environment that includes 15 mm Hg O_2, or more
- Initially, after 72 hours exposure to 1% oxygen, fibroblast proliferation increases by 71%
- During this period, fibroblast secretion of transforming growth factor (TGF)-β1

increases 9-fold, in turn causing upregulation of the procollagen gene.

This adaptation to hypoxia is only transient, and chronic oxygen deprivation severely diminishes fibroblast activity.[4] The surface of a poorly healing wound can be mapped with oxygen tension measurements, and fibroblast growth is progressively diminished until the hypoxic center of the lesion is reached, where proliferation is minimal or nil. By contrast, under hyperoxic conditions, fibroblasts are induced to differentiate into myofibroblasts, which are critical to wound closure through contraction.[17]

Epithelial

Numerous studies have shown that keratinocytes and fibroblasts migrate faster under hypoxic conditions.[18,19] Keratinocytes express more lamellipodia proteins and collagenase, and decrease lamellin-5 (motility brake) under hypoxia. This finding is expected, considering the mechanisms of natural dry wound healing, in which new skin regenerates underneath a stable eschar. The microenvironment through which the healing edge advances is protected from ambient oxygen, and the lack of blood vessels inside the eschar engender local hypoxia. In order for the epithelial edge to migrate the keratinocytes must carve a path through the tissue/eschar interface using collagenase and other enzymes.

Energy generation and use

Fundamental biochemical events such as molecular synthesis and transport cannot occur without a source of energy, and the ubiquitous source of energy in the human body is the coenzyme ATP. ATP is synthesized in mitochondria and stores chemical energy to fuel diverse biochemical processes in the body. The process by which ATP is created is known as oxidative phosphorylation and is critically dependent on the availability of molecular oxygen.[4] About 90% of the oxygen consumed by tissues goes to ATP synthesis.[5] Other energy stores generated through the citric acid cycle and the breakdown of fatty acids are also highly oxygen dependent.[7] The requirement for energy and, hence, the need for oxygen, is accentuated in healing tissue because cellular activities such as collagen synthesis, cell migration, and bacterial defense are heightened.

Influence of age

Another critical dimension to oxygen's role in healing relates to the age of the wounded host. The demographics of chronic nonhealing wounds indicate a strong relationship between incidence and advanced age, with most cases occurring in patients more than 60 years of age. Aging fibro-blasts show: [6,7,20]

- Reduced proliferative ability
- Diminished capacity to respond to growth factor stimulation
- Increased production of destructive enzymes such as MMPs.

Advanced age induces greater sensitivity to the negative effects of hypoxia. The migratory response of fibroblasts to TGF-β1 stimulation is blunted in older patients, compared with younger ones. Mustoe and colleagues[6] compared the effects of hypoxia on young (age 24–33 years) human dermal fibroblasts in tissue culture with fibroblasts from older (age 61–73 years) donors. Under 1% oxygen, there was greater decrease in TGF-β1 receptor expression in the aged cells (decrease of 12% in young fibroblasts vs 43% in old fibroblasts).

Responsiveness to TGF-β1 stimulation was reduced by advanced age:

- Activity of p42/p44 mitogen-activated kinase increased 50% in young cells versus decreasing 24% in the aged cells
- Unstimulated fibroblast migration increased 30% in young cells exposed to hypoxia, whereas the aged cells showed no change
- When TGF-β1 stimulation was added to the migration assay, young cells increased activity by 109% versus only 37% in the aged cells.[2]

Mendez and colleagues[20] studied fibroblasts harvested from the venous ulcer wound beds and used, as controls, cells taken from normal skin of the thigh.

- The 7 patients who were evaluated (mean age 51; range 36–67 years) had suffered wounds for a mean of 12.7 months (range 11–17 months)
- Chronic wound fibroblast growth rates were only one-third of those observed in the control cells ($P = .006$).

β-Galactosidase (β-GAL) activity was used as a sign of cellular senescence, a state of irreversible arrest of proliferation despite maintenance of metabolism.

- Six of 7 controls had no senescence associated (SA)-β-GAL activity
- All samples from the chronic wounds had measurable activity (mean 6.3%, median 2%)
- Level of SA-β-Gal correlated inversely with cellular growth rate ($R^2 = 0.77$).

The issue of cellular senescence may be more complex than mere chronologic age of the wounded patient. It may be the number of cell divisions that fibroblasts have undergone, rather than the age of the host, that defines the age of a cell. Many cell lines, including fibroblasts, are capable of only a finite number of cell divisions. Chronic wounds in young individuals may contain fibroblasts that have already reached the limit of their proliferative ability and are prematurely senescent.[7] Thus, although the lessons learned about the roles of oxygen in wound physiology are generally applicable, the degree to which patients may react to hypoxia and hyperoxia with the predicted responses may vary according to the physiologic age of the host cells.

Nitric oxide generation

Nitric oxide synthetase metabolizes the amino acid L-arginine into nitric oxide using oxygen as a substrate. Although nitric oxide is well known for its diverse, generally beneficial, effects on inflammation, angiogenesis, and cell proliferation, a full discussion of the putative benefits of enhanced nitric oxide is beyond the scope of this article.[21]

Role of Oxygen in Infection Control

During the initial phase of wound healing, activated leukocytes enter the wound and engulf bacteria. In the presence of adequate oxygen, an oxidative burst ensues, in which oxygen consumption increases as much as 50-fold compared with baseline conditions, and persists for hours, creating ROS that destroy the invaders.[22] ROS include:

- Peroxide anion (HO_2^-)
- Hydroxyl ion (OH^-)
- Superoxide anion (O_2^-)
- Hydrogen peroxide (H_2O_2).

About 98% of oxygen consumption by leukocytes is related to this respiratory burst, which is facilitated by phagocyte (neutrophil, eosinophil, monocyte, and macrophage) cell membrane–bound nicotinamide adenine dinucleotide phosphate (NADPH) oxidase[23]:

$$NADPH + 2O_2 \rightarrow NADP + 2O_2^- + H^+$$

Glucose provides the energy to drive the reaction, generating substantial amounts of lactate in the process.[1]

ROS, and especially superoxide, are toxic and kill bacteria, then are rapidly degraded to H_2O_2 and other by-products.[10,24] The kinetics are such that the killing process works at 50% of maximal speed in the presence of oxygen at 40 to 80 mm Hg, and as much as 400 mm Hg are required to increase the velocity to 90%.[4] Neutrophils therefore lose most of their ability to kill bacteria at less than 40 mm Hg.[7] Patients afflicted with chronic granulomatous disease, which is characterized by defects in the genes that encode NADPH oxidase, have increased susceptibility to infection, and also show impaired wound healing.[10]

The results of many investigations suggest that, in a reduced P_{O_2} wound environment, the ability of leukocytes to generate ROS is substantially impaired, and therefore the ability to ward off colonization/infection is lowered. In vitro studies of leukocytes obtained from venous blood show that neutrophil oxygen consumption increases as ambient oxygen concentration increases, and suggest that increasing ambient oxygen to more than physiologic levels may induce even greater ROS synthesis. However, there is the theoretic potential that excess ROS may be destructive and counterproductive to wound healing. The body has a robust system for removal of ROS by superoxide dismutase, catalase, and reduced glutathione, and the wound concentration of ROS is the net result of synthesis and destruction. ROS clearance requires an adequate circulatory supply.[25]

The potential to increase local wound oxygenation to supraphysiologic levels and cure or prevent infection was evaluated in 30 patients with chronic diabetic wounds. Patients were randomized to receive standard care (wound dressings; antibiotics guided by culture results) alone or in combination with 4 hyperbaric oxygen therapy (HBOT) treatments given during a 2-week period. In the control group, cultures grew significant colony counts of 16 different isolates at baseline, and 12 at the end of the observation period; in the patients receiving HBOT, isolates were reduced from 19 before treatment to only 3 afterward ($P<.05$). HBOT seemed particularly effective in controlling *Pseudomonas* and *Escherichia coli*. Seven patients in the control group required major lower extremity amputation (5 for spreading infection) versus 2 in the HBOT-treated patients ($P<.05$).[26]

Redox Signaling

The traditional view of ROS has been that they are destructive to bacteria and host cells, necessary for wound hygiene in the early phase of healing, but otherwise counterproductive to the normal healing cascade.[12] This view has prompted numerous clinical trials testing the role of various antioxidants in ameliorating different disease conditions, and these trials typically have shown disappointing results.[27–29]

The late 1990s brought a growing appreciation that, at very low levels, ROS (particularly H_2O_2) serve as signaling messengers, a role independent of bacterial killing.[10] NADPH oxidase exists not only in neutrophils but also in nonphagocytic wound cell lines, and there is a continuous low-level production of ROS that is unrelated to leukocytes, oxidative burst, or response to wound colonization or debris.[30] ROS bind to proteins and can alter their conformation, leading to increases or decreases in their functional abilities.[31] H_2O_2 functions primarily by oxidizing cysteine moieties. The molecule has a potent effect in recruiting leukocytes to the wound site, and the concentration of endogenous hydrogen peroxide increases significantly at the wound margins within the first few minutes of injury. The functions of important growth factors such as VEGF, platelet-derived growth factor (PDGF), keratinocyte growth factor (KGF), and TGF-α are inhibited in the absence of such signals.[32] Thus, overexpression of catalase, which removes H_2O_2 from the wound, is associated with impaired angiogenesis and delayed wound closure.[33] Cellular functions like migration and leukocyte recruitment are also inhibited in the absence of H_2O_2.[12] Micromolar levels of peroxide can be measured in normal wound fluid.[34] Research in oncology indicates that low-level ROS foster angiogenesis, and overexpression of extracellular super oxide dismutase inhibits tumor vascularization in mice.

Note

The low physiologic concentration of H_2O_2 must be distinguished from the 3% v/v strength that is available commercially and often used to clean and disinfect wounds; at such high concentrations, severe oxidative damage to wounds is noted, and this is contraindicated in modern wound management. However, at 0.15% H_2O_2, topical angiogenesis is favorably influenced.[31]

The state of overabundance or underabundance of ROS is reflected in the redox potential of the wound microenvironment. The ratio of NADH to NAD^+ has been used as a redox index, and transcription of various genes important in wound repair seems to be responsive to this ratio. Every phase of the wound healing cascade (hemostasis, inflammation, proliferation, epithelialization) has been shown to have key steps that require NADPH oxidase action.[24] Individuals with mutations in either p47[phox] or Rac2, which are each associated with action of this enzyme, show impaired wound healing.

Hypoxia

Many of our conclusions about the role of oxygen in wound repair come from observations of the defects in healing that are associated with hypoxia. Absolute hypoxia is usually defined as an oxygen level less than 30 mm Hg.[2] However, hypoxia is more typically a relative term, indicating insufficient oxygen for the tissue and physiologic situation under consideration.[12] For example, with infection or an open wound, oxygen demand increases and levels of delivery that might be adequate for intact, uninfected dermis may be deficient. Cells challenged with hypoxia must reduce activity and rely on anaerobic metabolism, or die. Acute and mild/moderate hypoxia usually leads to cellular adaptation and survival; prolonged and more extreme hypoxia may result in cellular death.

Hypoxia is a more frequent issue in wound repair than is commonly appreciated. Wound bed oxygenation depends on:

- Pulmonary uptake
- Hemoglobin level
- Cardiac output
- Vascular patency
- Capillary density
- Factors that deplete oxygen such as parenchymal consumption and inflammatory cell activity.

Decreased wound oxygen tension occurs not only from macrocirculatory issues but also because oxygen is consumed by metabolically active and proliferative cells located along the path from capillaries to the healing edge of tissue **Box 2**. As much as a 150-μm distance from the nearest capillary to the healing edge may need to be nourished by oxygen diffusion.[4] This effect is magnified in the presence of heavy bacterial colonization or infection, further consuming oxygen and decreasing the available oxygen to the healing wound. A vicious cycle may ensue in which bacterial oxygen consumption reduces the ability of leukocytes to synthesize ROS, enabling further bacterial proliferation, and so on. The centers of even seemingly well-oxygenated wounds may be hypoxic because of high oxygen extraction along the path of diffusion from capillaries.[7] Although circulating blood may contain a Po_2 of 100 mm Hg, the periphery of a dermal wound may be

60 mm Hg and, at the center of the wound, readings can be as low as 0 to 10 mm Hg.[1,35] Many chronic wounds suffer local hypoxia; in one study, normal, nonwounded tissue showed oxygen tensions of 30 to 50 mm Hg, whereas measurements of Po_2 in nonhealing chronic wounds in the same patients were in the range of 5 to 20 mm Hg.[4]

At present, it is not easy to reconcile all the scientific knowledge about effects of hypoxia and hyperoxia on wound tissues and to synthesize all the evidence into a coherent story.[19] Hypoxia has been traditionally regarded as an important stimulus to fibroblast growth and angiogenesis. Hypoxia encourages angiogenesis by increasing levels of hypoxia-inducible factor 1 (HIF-1), which in turn binds to the promoter segment of the VEGF gene and activates transcription, leading to higher synthesis of VEGF, the principal angiogenetic growth factor in human physiology.[2,7] Paradoxically, multiple studies have shown that hyperoxic conditions induce greater angiogenesis, perhaps by increasing local ROS.[32,36]

Acute hypoxia induces temporary increases in cellular replication (3-fold increase under 5 mm Hg compared with 150 mm Hg). This has been associated with a 6.3-fold increase in the expression of TGF-β1 and enhanced procollagen synthesis.[7] However, these increases in proliferation and metabolic activity are short lived and, when these conditions are maintained for more than a week, cellular growth and synthetic activity decrease to significantly less than baseline physiologic levels.[16] The situation is reversible; restoration of normal oxygen levels restores typical proliferation rates, and a second bout of hypoxia induces a second temporary burst of fibroblast activity. In chronic hypoxia, the production and secretion of the most important cytokines and chemokines central to healing (including TNF-α, TGF-α, TGF-β1, KGF, EGF, PDFG, and insulin growth factor) require oxygen and are reduced or absent.

There seem to be at least 2 ways to reconcile the older concept that hypoxia is beneficial with modern understanding that healing proceeds more quickly with increased oxygen delivery.

1. The true primary stimulus to VEGF secretion, angiogenesis and collagen deposition may be lactate, more than hypoxia.[4,5] Even in well-perfused and properly oxygenated wounds, lactate may accumulate because leukocytes, fibroblasts, and endothelial cells lack mitochondria and rely on anaerobic glycolysis for energy production; a principal by-product of this glycolysis is lactate.[1] Thus, lactate levels may still be increased in hyperoxia, albeit less so compared with hypoxia.

Box 2
Clinical pearl: wound hypoxia

Clinical pearl: wound hypoxia is under-recognized and may occur in even normally perfused lesions because of high oxygen extraction along the diffusion path from the feeding capillary to the edge of healing tissue.

2. It is possible that the P_{O_2} gradient between the capillary and the most distant cell may drive angiogenesis more than the absolute level of P_{O_2}. The immediate effect of hyperoxygenation of the blood may be to increase this gradient, and increased oxygen diffusion to areas of low P_{O_2} may follow.

Therapeutic Oxygen Supplementation

Because of the high incidence of wound hypoxia and the knowledge of the deleterious effects of inadequate oxygen on healing, it is natural to consider the potential of oxygen supplementation to improve wound repair **Box 3**. In some instances, the most effective way to improve wound oxygenation may involve measures to enhance blood flow rather than changing the oxygen content of the blood. Such maneuvers may include hydration and relief of vasoconstriction using local warmth and analgesics. Because hemoglobin is nearly saturated in most individuals, enhancing inspired oxygen may only modestly increase peripheral delivery. Other techniques for hyperoxygenation of wounds include breathing oxygen under supranormal pressures (hyperbaric oxygen [HBO]) or bathing the wound topically with an enhanced oxygen environment (topical oxygen therapy [TOT]). The remainder of this article focuses on various attempts to supplement oxygen for the benefit of healing acute and chronic wounds.

Enriched inhaled oxygen to prevent surgical site infections

Under normal circumstances, hemoglobin is almost completely saturated while breathing room air under normobaric conditions, so the opportunity for increased oxygen delivery with enhanced forced inspiratory oxygen (FiO_2) is limited. However, by increasing the serum P_{O_2}, the tissue diffusion gradient is increased. For example, in the rabbit ischemic ear model, breathing 100% O_2 at 1 ATA increases blood P_{O_2} from 90 to 450 mm Hg. At less than 20% O_2, most of the oxygen is consumed within 70 μm of the nourishing capillary, but, after

breathing 100% O_2 for 45 minutes, there is measureable increase in P_{O_2} even 150 μm away.[5]

Knighton and colleagues[37] in 1984 showed that higher inspired concentrations of oxygen lowered the extent of infection induced by intradermal injection of bacteria. Guinea pigs were given intradermal injections containing 10^8 E coli, then were treated with either 12%, 21%, or 45% inhaled normobaric oxygen. The end point, the size of the resulting lesion, was substantially reduced with increased oxygen ($P<.005$ for either 21% or 45% vs 12%; $P<.01$ for 45% vs 21%). The therapeutic effect was attributed to improved leukocyte killing with higher oxygen tension.

Conversely, it has been noted that the rate of surgical site infection (SSI) in surgical patients increases as systemic subcutaneous oxygen tension decreases.[38]

- Upper arm subcutaneous P_{O_2} measurements were conducted in 130 patients who underwent major general surgery (mostly abdominal) on the day of surgery and during postoperative days 1 and 2
- A total of 24 patients developed infection at the surgical site
- There was a strong correlation between decreased P_{O_2} and the development of infection ($r = 0.91$; $P<.001$).

The potential for supplemental inspired oxygen to lower the rate of SSI has been studied extensively. Grief and colleagues[39] randomized 500 adult patients undergoing colorectal resection to breathe 30% or 80% oxygen during, and for 2 hours after, the procedure. After surgery, patients were evaluated daily until hospital discharge, and then in the clinic 2 weeks later. Although the anesthesiologists knew the treatment to which each patient was randomized, the surgeon conducting the operation and the postoperative evaluation was blinded to this assignment. Wounds were considered infected if there were clinical signs and symptoms of infection, and if fluid or pus expressed from the wound cultured positive.

- Thirteen patients in the 80% oxygen group developed wound infection versus 28 patients in the 30% group (5.2% vs 11.2%; $P = .01$)
- Six patients in the 30% group had signs of infection but cultured negative, compared with 4 in the 80% group.

The investigators concluded that supplemental inspired oxygen was effective in lowering the perioperative wound infection rate.

Box 3
Clinical pearl: wound open to breathe

Clinical pearl: leaving a wound open to breathe

I wish I had a penny for every time I have explained to patients and families that wounds do not breathe! Under normobaric room air conditions, all the oxygen delivery to a wound is internal, and wounds can (and generally should) be occluded to maintain a moist wound environment and exclude dirt.

A similar prospective, randomized trial of 30% versus 80% inspired oxygen was conducted by Belda and colleagues.[40]

- Three hundred patients were randomized to yield 291 who were evaluable
- The rate of SSI was unusually high (57 patients [39.3%]) and there was no clear explanation for this finding
- The incidence of SSI was reduced significantly in response to higher inspired oxygen: 24% versus 15% infected for patients treated with 30% and 80% oxygen, respectively ($P = .04$).

Chura and colleagues[41] reviewed the literature and conducted a meta-analysis on the value of supplemental oxygen in preventing SSI in colorectal surgery. Among thousands of articles that emerged from a keyword search on "surgical site infection" and "perioperative oxygen" only 4 studies met criteria for sufficient scientific rigor to warrant analysis. Although there was significant heterogeneity among these studies, the investigators concluded that there was sufficient evidence to support the assertion that perioperative oxygen supplementation reduces SSI. The aggregate number of patients in these studies was 943 (477 who received supplemental O_2 and 466 who were controls). The pooled relative risk for SSI with perioperative O_2 supplementation was 0.68 (95% confidence interval, 0.49 to 0.94).

Only 1 major study failed to show reduction of SSI with supplemental oxygen. Meyhoff and colleagues[42] studied 1400 Danish patients undergoing laparotomy at 14 hospitals. Patients and observers were blinded to the random assignment to 30% or 80% O_2. The study end point was superficial or deep wound infection, or intra-abdominal infection, using the Centers for Disease Control and Prevention definitions. The low-oxygen group had an SSI rate of 20.1% versus 19.1% for 80% O_2 (not significant [NS]). Most patients received perioperative antibiotic prophylaxis with cefuroxime and metronidazole or benzyl-penicillin and gentamycin; perhaps this accounts for the apparently discrepancy between this study and the others cited earlier.

On balance, it seems that increasing the concentration of inhaled oxygen is likely of benefit. In 2008, the UK National Institute for Health and Clinical Excellence concluded that, "The mechanism for improved blood oxygen carriage due to increased FiO_2 is physiologically not clear. However, this simple, cheap intervention deserves further investigation."[43]

Systemic HBOT

HBOT is conducted in single-person or multiple-person chambers that completely envelop patients in an environment of 2 to 2.5 atmospheres (atm) and 100% oxygen.[44] Sessions are typically delivered for 90 to 120 minutes daily (sometimes twice daily), and therapeutic courses lasting 2 to 8 weeks are typical. Because most patients under room air conditions show hemoglobin oxygen saturations of 90% or greater, the incremental binding of oxygen to hemoglobin induced by HBOT is marginal. However, independently of the normal mechanism of oxygen transport to tissues via hemoglobin binding, HBOT dissolves substantial amounts of oxygen directly into serum, much as carbon dioxide is dissolved under pressure into carbonated beverages.

- Serum Po_2 can reach 1200 to 2000 mm Hg during treatment sessions.[35]
- Total blood oxygen content, which is ordinarily in the range of 20 volume %, increases to about 27 volume % during 100% oxygen breathing at 3 ATA pressure.
- Because oxygen delivery from capillaries into tissue is driven by diffusion along a gradient, large increases of capillary Po_2 result in substantial increases in oxygenation at the cellular level. When the Po_2 is increased to 2000 mm Hg, oxygen may diffuse as far as 246 μm.
- As shown by the classic report of Boerema and colleagues[45] in 1960, sufficient oxygen can be dissolved in the bloodstream to maintain life and vital organ function even in the absence of hemoglobin.
- Following a session of HBOT, skin oxygen tension remains increased for a period of 30 minutes to 4 hours.

The details of nearly 400 years of hyperbaric medicine have been described by Kindwall.[46] The history of HBOT is checkered. On a naïve level, hyperoxygenation of tissue seems to be potentially beneficial in a wide variety of pathologic conditions. Given the sensitivity of peripheral and central nervous tissue to hypoxia, for example, HBOT has been attempted in a range of neurologic diseases and conditions. In past decades, hyperbaric operating rooms were used to conduct procedures such as carotid endarterectomy, in which temporary brain ischemia was anticipated. In general, results of HBOT for these and many other conditions were disappointing.

The combination of overly optimistic expectations and disappointing outcomes led to the perception that HBOT was not useful in any medical condition, and the therapy was relegated to the realm of quackery in the opinion of many practitioners since the 1970s. Nevertheless, an increase in interest and effort to understand the physiology of wound healing in the past 20 years has generated a large body of evidence both in favor of the results of HBOT and to explain the mechanisms by which HBOT is beneficial. Thus, opinion has returned to a middle ground in which HBOT is understood to be a valuable adjunctive wound healing therapy but not a panacea. Nevertheless there are still skeptics of HBOT who think that, for most patients, the therapy is unnecessary and that oxygenation of most wounds can be achieved in other ways, such as by improving local perfusion.[1]

HBOT: growing scientific basis

Medical societies, government agencies, and health insurers now agree that there is a legitimate role for HBOT in a variety of conditions, including many aspects of chronic open wounds. The American Diabetes Association endorsed HBOT for treating recalcitrant diabetic foot ulcers in 1999; 3 years later, the Centers for Medicare and Medicaid Services announced its concurrence and its policy to reimburse for such treatments in patients who had failed to heal with a month of standard care.[14] Professional societies such as the Undersea and Hyperbaric Medical Society and the Wound Healing Society have included adjunctive HBOT in suggested algorithms of care for diabetic foot ulceration.

There is a large and growing body of scientific information to indicate the potential physiologic benefits of HBOT in wound healing. Typical HBOT increases Po_2 to 1200 mm Hg and increases O_2 diffusion distance from 60 to 250 μm.[47] Fibroblast proliferation is improved by this treatment. Hehenberger and colleagues[22] described a series of experiments in which fibroblasts harvested from normal patients undergoing reduction mammoplasty were compared with cells derived from specimens of diabetic foot ulcer beds. Cells were plated in tissue culture medium and placed inside a monoplace hyperbaric oxygen (HBO) chamber, then subjected to air (as control, at 795 and 1875 mm Hg) and 100% oxygen at various pressures from 795 to 2250 mm Hg. Total cell count was determined by measuring DNA content in the specimens immediately before treatment and after 24 hours. Although pressurized air did not induce fibroblast growth, fibroblasts proliferated more as Po_2 was increased, and maximal proliferation rate was observed at 1875 mm Hg (2.4 ATA).[22] HBOT was able to restore fibroblast growth in diabetic ulcer cells to the level seen in the normal control cells. Other investigators have noted that HBOT induces fibroblasts to differentiate into myofibroblasts, which are responsible for wound contraction.[48]

See **Box 4** for a summary of HBOT wound healing indications.

HBOT treatment and wound vascularity

A common observation among hyperbaric physicians is the large increase in wound vascularity after patients are treated for several weeks. HBOT has been shown to increase VEGF mRNA levels in endothelial cells and macrophages, and increased VEGF is noted in wound fluid of patients receiving this treatment.[7] Much of this effect may be mediated by increased nitric oxide.[49,50] HBOT induces endothelial progenitor cells (EPCs) to migrate out of bone marrow, circulate, and settle in the peripheral wound, forming vascular buds.[51,52] Circulating EPCs in the peripheral blood are diminished in diabetes mellitus; HBOT reverses this. The HBOT-induced steep oxygen gradient between capillary and hypoxic wound bed prompts macrophage migration and release of angiogenetic growth factors. There is a distinction between angiogenesis (proliferation and migration of resident endothelial cells supported by fibroblasts) and vasculogenesis (a de novo process whereby EPCs enter a wound, differentiate into endothelial cells, and create a new vascular network). HBOT facilitates both these regenerative processes by increasing wound VEGF, basic fibroblast growth factor, and TGF-β1. Patients undergoing 20 HBO treatments in preparation for dental procedures related to osteoradionecrosis of the mandible were found to have a 5-fold increase in EPCs. Under inhibition of nitric oxide synthetase, this effect is blocked. Maximal stimulation of peripheral nitric oxide synthetase requires up to 2.8 ATA.[12]

HBOT and hypoxia/hyperoxia

We have noted that both hypoxia and hyperoxia have certain salutary effects on healing. Perhaps

---

Box 4
Generally accepted wound-related indications for HBOT

- Necrotizing soft tissue infections
- Radiation damage to soft tissue and/or bone
- Moderate and deep diabetic foot and leg wounds
- Crush injury
- Gas gangrene

by fortune more than design, the current regimen of HBOT makes use of both stimuli: during HBO treatment, and for about 4 hours afterward, the supplemental oxygen facilitates fibroblast growth and collagen deposition and maturation, whereas during the remaining 20 hours before the next treatment, relative hypoxia stimulates angiogenesis.

HBOT and antibiotics

HBOT also increases the susceptibility of various bacteria to antibiotics, but is this strain specific and the effect cannot be generalized to all pathogens, whether aerobic or anaerobic.[5,7]

HBOT and MMPs

Sander and colleagues[36] used a model of impaired healing created by depleting mice of macrophages to study the effects of HBOT. Healing was restored to normal pace in HBOT-treated animals, even though the wounds were not ischemic or hypoxic. The author proposed that the benefit of HBOT was mediated through contradictory effects on MMPs. The activity of tissue inhibitor of metalloproteinase-1 (TIMP-1) was increased by the treatment. However, HBOT increased TNF-α in the wound bed, which typically increases the supply of MMPs available for selective tissue breakdown necessary for neovascularization and epithelial migration.[36]

HBOT and granulation tissue

In the rabbit ischemic ear model, HBOT increased granulation tissue and epithelial regrowth; the response was accentuated when growth factors were added to the HBOT.[53] Two of the 3 arteries supplying the external ear were ligated to create tissue ischemia, then 6-mm, full-thickness dermal wounds were created (n = 42). Wounds were treated with PDGF-BB, TGF-β1, or buffered saline; animals underwent HBO for 90 min/d at 1, 2, or 3 ATA 100% O_2 for up to a week. Treatment at 1 ATA did not alter epithelial advance or granulation tissue. Hyperoxygenation at 2 and 3 ATA increased granulation and increased wound Po_2 to as high as 300 mm Hg, increasing tissue volume by 100% (P = .03) but not influencing epithelial advance.[54] In combination with topical growth factors, granulation tissue increased by 200% (P = .0001) and epithelial advance increased significantly.

Obstacles to defining benefits of HBOT

A major obstacle to precise definition of the benefits of HBOT is the paucity of scientifically rigorous clinical studies. In 2005, Roeckl-Wiedmann and colleagues[55] performed an extensive search through some 24 electronic databases as well as a manual search through texts to gather 78 articles that purportedly offered clinical evidence on the role of HBOT in wound management. Of these, only 21 were deemed to be suitable human clinical trials, and 15 were excluded because they were not randomized, not clearly focused on 1 wound cause, used TOT instead of HBOT, or reported data that had already been published elsewhere. Six publications of at least moderate scientific merit were left: 5 on diabetic foot ulcers and 1 on venous leg ulcers.

Kessler and colleagues' study on diabetic foot ulcers

Kessler and colleagues[56] noted that HBOT doubled the rate of wound healing (P = .037) compared with controls during 2 weeks of treatment, but, once the twice-daily HBOT treatments were discontinued, the rate of healing in the control and HBOT groups equalized.[56] Twenty-eight patients were randomized, 15 to HBOT and 13 to control therapy, including off-loading. Patients were excluded if they suffered significant arterial occlusive disease or serious contraindications to HBOT (emphysema, claustrophobia, proliferating retinopathy). The groups were similar in terms of demographic factors and indicators of diabetic complications (renal, ocular, vascular), and all suffered with neuropathy. Lesions ranged from Wagner grade I to III. HBOT was delivered as 100% oxygen at 2.5 ATA pressure, giving two 5-minute air breaks during each treatment session. Only 1 patient had barotrauma to the ear and had to discontinue participation. Peri-wound TcPo2 increased from a mean of 22 to 454 mm Hg with first treatment, and 26 to 550 mm Hg after 20 treatments (P<.001). At day 15 (completion of HBOT), the surface area of ulcers treated with HBOT was reduced substantially more than the healing that was observed in control subjects (41.8%±25.5% surface area reduction with HBOT vs 21.7% ± 27.3% in controls; P = .037). By day 30, the control group had caught up: respective surface area reductions were 48.1% (±30.3%) and 41.7% (±27.3%; NS).

Faglia and colleagues' study on ischemic diabetic wounds

HBOT reduced lower amputation rates significantly in patients with ischemic diabetic wounds.[57] Seventy diabetic patients who were hospitalized for severe foot wounds were considered appropriate candidates for HBOT. They consented to randomization to standard therapy with or without HBOT. Two patients dropped out (1 died of a stroke shortly after hospital admission; the other withdrew consent for treatment). Of the remaining patients, 35 underwent HBOT and 33 did not. There were no differences in the treatment groups in terms of demographic features, depth of foot ulceration, other diabetic complications, circulatory status, or duration of hospitalization. In the treatment groups, Wagner grade III and IV lesions predominated (25.7% and 62.8% in the HBOT group, and 24.2% and 60.6% in the control groups, respectively). All patients underwent an initial aggressive excisional debridement shortly after admission to the hospital, then twice-daily dressing changes and antibiotics guided by frequent wound cultures. Patients receiving HBOT received an average of 38 treatments; daily in the beginning and then 5 days per week later on (2.5 ATA 100% O_2, 90 minutes). The end point of the study was the incidence of major amputation. Three patients receiving HBOT required below-knee or above-knee amputations, compared with 11 controls (8.6% vs 33.3%, respectively; $P = .016$). $TcPo_2$ measurements were included in the study: at baseline the 2 patient groups had similar readings (23.2±10.7 mm Hg vs 21.3±10.7 mm Hg, respectively; NS). However, at hospital discharge, the values had increased to 37.3 (±16.1) mm Hg and 26.3 (±13.5) mm Hg, respectively. The greater improvement in the HBOT group was highly statistically significant ($P = .0002$). The investigators concluded that the enhanced increase in $TcPo_2$ was related to improved angiogenesis in and around the wound, and they proposed that HBOT is effective in lowering the incidence of major amputation in diabetic wounds.

Baroni and colleagues' study on diabetic foot ulcers

Baroni and colleagues[58] conducted a nonrandomized comparison of the outcomes of 18 hospitalized patients with diabetic foot ulcers treated with standard of care plus HBOT with another group of 10 patients treated identically but without HBOT. All patients had advanced diabetes, and most suffered retinopathy, neuropathy, and vascular occlusive disease. In the HBOT group, 16 patients healed versus 1 in the comparator group ($P = .001$). Two patients receiving HBOT and 4 comparator patients underwent amputation. The investigators concluded that there is major benefit in HBOT for amputation avoidance.

Abidia and colleagues' study on ischemic lower extremity ulcers

Abidia and colleagues[59] conducted a small double-blind study in which patients with ischemic lower extremity ulcers were randomized to hyperbaric air or hyperbaric oxygen treatment. By 6 weeks, 5 of 8 wounds healed in the oxygen group versus 1 of 8 of the controls (NS because of small numbers). At 1 year, all the HBOT wounds remained healed but the wound that had healed in the control group reopened, and the difference in 1-year closure was significantly better in the treated group ($P = .026$). The investigators analyzed overall direct patient treatment costs (fees for dressings, clinic visits, and hospitalizations) and found that HBOT was also able to show cost-effectiveness (based on 100 UK pounds per HBO treatment session). At 6 weeks, median wound surface area closure was 100% in the HBOT group and 52% in controls ($P = .027$). Although the study included few patients, the randomization was strict and the methodology was rigorous.

Kranke and colleagues' study on diabetic foot ulcers

Kranke and colleagues[60] found only 5 publications that met the standards for inclusion in a Cochrane Review of the evidence in favor of HBOT for chronic wounds. The investigators concluded that HBOT significantly reduces the chance of amputation and may increase the chance of healing at 1 year for diabetic foot ulcers. However, they concluded that there is a need for further substantiation because the number of patients on which these conclusions were based is small, and the trial methodologies imperfect. They could not justify the use of HBOT in the management of other wound causes based on current evidence. The report estimated that 4 diabetic ulcers needed to be treated with HBOT to prevent 1 amputation.

Lin and colleagues' study on diabetic foot lesions

Lin and colleagues[61] randomized 29 patients with Wagner 0, 1, and 2 foot lesions to standard care with and without HBOT. Although patients started the study with similar values, after 30 HBO treatments, the patients receiving HBOT had significantly reduced HgA1c (6.6±1.7 vs 9.3±4.3) $TcPo_2$ (57.5±20.7 vs 35.8±21.2), and laser Doppler perfusion scan flux (35.6±7.0 vs 25.8±4.1; all 3 comparisons were statistically significant at the $P<.05$ level).

Predictive ability in HBOT

A frequent objection to HBOT is the inability to predict accurately which patients will receive benefit. Because there are certain indications that sometimes have good responses, patients are usually treated empirically for several weeks, assessed for response, and then continued or terminated according to clinical parameters. Perhaps because of well-intentioned optimism, many patients are treated for weeks or even months, at great expense ($1000 per treatment at our center) but with minimal tangible improvement. Fife and colleagues[34] found only moderate predictive ability of $TcPo_2$ to distinguish patients who would benefit from HBOT, whether measured under room air, breathing 100% oxygen at sea level, or in the chamber. Barnes[47] noted that, for diabetic lesions, the extent of the wound according to the Wagner scale correlated well with response to HBOT, with Wagner 3, 4, and 5 lesions responding well 77%, 64%, and 30% of the time, respectively. In the same report, patients who achieve a periwound $TcPo_2$ of 200 while breathing 100% oxygen at 2.5 ATA were likely to heal.

Complications in HBOT

HBOT generally is safe and comfortable; nevertheless, there are well-known complications that may occur. One set of risks relates to maintaining the patient under supranormal external pressure. About 60% to 70% of patients experience measureable, but reversible, myopia; patients with presbyopia may experience temporary improvement in visual acuity during the course of therapy. The incidence of otic barotrauma has been quoted between about 2% and 20%.[35,47,55] In my experience, the incidence is even higher, and fully one-quarter of my patients require temporary tympanostomy tubes to equalize pressures in the middle ear and prevent permanent damage. The tubes are easily removed (or sometimes fall out spontaneously) and the tympanic membranes typically heal within days afterward. Other barotrauma is less frequent; the incidence of pneumothorax has been cited at 1 in 1 million treatments. HBOT imposes increased afterload on the left ventricle and patients with New York Heart Association class 3 and 4 congestive heart failure, with ejection fraction less than 35%, should not be treated, because their cardiac situation may worsen.

The other set of potential complications relates to the effects of oxygen as a medicine. Perhaps the most feared complication is oxygen toxicity seizure, the risk of which is about 0.01% to 0.03%. These seizures, which are usually over within the brief time it takes to switch the breathing mixture from 100% to air and to decompress the HBO chamber, do not cause permanent brain damage and are random events that do not necessarily preclude further HBOT. Regimens dictating a 90-minute treatment and limiting pressure to about 2.5 ATA are based on known tolerance of patients to high levels of oxygen for given periods of time. The risk of seizure may be lowered by giving a 5-minute period of air breathing, rather than 100% oxygen, every half hour while in the chamber. There are other theoretic risks of excessive oxygen, such as pulmonary toxicity and of enhancing tumor growth, but these have not been borne out in everyday practice.

Indications for HBOT

At present, the generally approved wound-related indications for HBOT include moderate and deep diabetic foot/leg lesions, necrotizing soft tissue infections, radiation damage to soft tissue and/or bone (osteoradionecrosis), selected problem wounds (**Figs. 1** and **2**), compromised skin grafts and flaps, crush injury, clostridial myositis, gas gangrene, and refractory osteomyelitis. Perioperative treatments have been particularly useful in patients with osteoradionecrosis of the mandible who are undergoing dental extractions or implants; typical regimens call for 10 preoperative treatments and then postprocedure treatment until full healing is observed. Similarly, in anticipation of skin grafts or flaps that may be compromised because of tension or because the tissue to be closed has previously been irradiated, a brief period of preoperative treatment followed by resumption of HBOT as soon as practical after surgery optimizes graft/flap take.

The American Diabetes Association has since 1999 endorsed the used of HBOT as an adjunctive therapy for severe diabetic wounds that fail to respond to standard therapy.[14] The Centers for Medicare and Medicaid Services in 2002 approved the therapy for treatment Wagner III to IV ulcers. Professional organizations such as the Undersea and Hyperbaric Medical Society and Wound Healing Society have included HBOT in their suggested algorithms of care. More than 90% of wounds closed with HBOT remain healed 4 years later. Although health economic aspects of treatment are beyond the scope of this article, a case can be made that the expense of HBOT is justifiable with cost-effectiveness data.[47]

TOT

TOT involves enclosing a body part (usually an extremity) in a portable chamber that circulates pure oxygen over the wound surface. Potential advantages to this approach, compared with HBOT, include lower cost, greater convenience, therapy not limited to 2 hours per day, and success not dependent on the macrocirculation and microcirculation to the wound bed.[7] Potential complications of HBOT, such as oxygen toxicity to tissues/organs, may be avoided by using TOT.[35]

TOT Penetration of Wound Surface

Perhaps the most controversial issue is the ability of TOT to achieve meaningful penetration of the

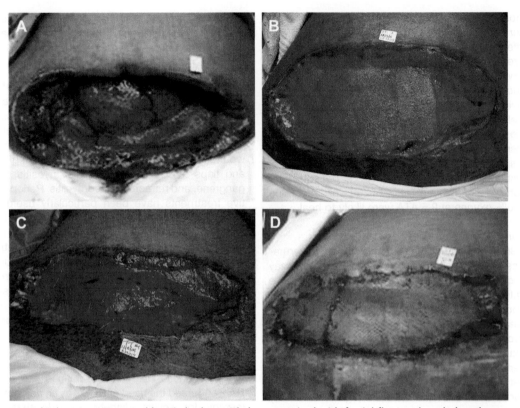

Fig. 1. Multiple-recurrent ventral hernia had recently been repaired with fascial flaps and mesh, but the wound became infected and dehisced shortly after surgery. The patient was returned to surgery and the mesh was removed. (*A*) Exposed abdominal organs thinly covered with collagen mesh. (*B*) After 20 HBO treatments, there is substantial in-growth of vessels and soft tissue. (*C*) After nearly 40 HBO treatments, the wound has partially contracted and the soft tissue coverage has thickened. (*D*) Perioperative HBOT was used to support the take of partial-thickness skin grafts, achieving definitive closure of the wound.

wound surface and reach the cells/tissues that would benefit from hyperoxygenation. This issue has been addressed both with direct measurement of tissue oxygen levels and, indirectly, by showing the biochemical and biologic effects of TOT. Fries and colleagues[35] showed that, at a depth of 2 mm into the wound bed, P_{O_2} increased from its baseline of 5 to 7 mm Hg to 40 mm Hg

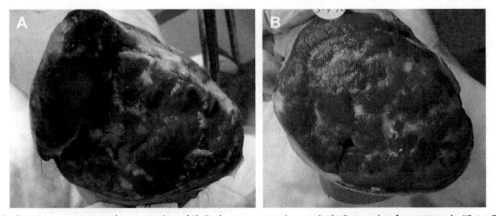

Fig. 2. Open transmetatarsal amputation. (*A*) Early postoperative period. Cut ends of metatarsals #2 to 5 are exposed. (*B*) After approximately 40 HBO treatments. Bone ends are covered. Healthy granulation tissue fills the wound.

after 4 minutes of TOT. Standardized full-thickness wounds on the backs of pigs were treated with either topical air or topical pure oxygen. By the second day of treatment, the surface area of the oxygen wounds was significantly ($P<.05$) reduced compared with the controls, and the acceleration in healing was maintained to 3 weeks ($P<.005$). Healed wounds were subjected to 3-mm punch biopsy and histologic evaluation; TOT wounds were more mature than the controls, in terms of epithelial architecture, expression of keratin-14, and expression of VEGF and α-smooth muscle actin. Under resting conditions, wound site tissue Po_2 levels were 4 times higher in the TOT versus the control wounds (42 vs 11 mm Hg; $P<.05$).

In another report, db/db diabetic obese mice were subjected to standardized full-thickness wounds and then randomized to TOT or control dressings.[62] TOT was delivered as pure oxygen at low flow (3 mL/h) over the wounds. The surface area of the TOT wounds was significantly smaller at 6 and 10 days ($P = .022$ and $P = .008$, respectively). Histologic sections of the wounds showed more extensive collagen deposition in the TOT-treated lesions.

TOT and Increased VEGF

Gordillo and colleagues[63] showed that TOT increased VEGF up to 20-fold in diabetic foot ulcers. A large clinic population was screened to enroll 57 patients who suffered a variety of chronic wounds. The criteria by which these patients were selected were not described in detail. These patients were assessed for HBOT but patients who had contraindications were offered TOT; this yielded a population of 32 HBO-treated and 25 TOT-treated patients. Patients who consented to serial biopsies underwent wound edge biopsy just before initiation of treatment and again at 7 and 14 weeks into therapy. Tissue levels of mRNA expressed by the genes for VEGF, TGF-β1, and COLIA1 were measured. In patients who experienced complete wound healing, VEGF expression was substantially increased by TOT but not by HBOT; expression of the other 2 genes did not show a significant difference with either treatment. The issues with study design limit the interpretation of these results, but demonstration of increased VEGF expression implied that TOT succeeded in penetrating the wound with oxygen to a meaningful extent.

TOT Versus Silver Alginate

Blackman and colleagues[64] conducted a prospective, but not randomized, comparison of patients treated with TOT versus a silver alginate dressing.

TOT treatments were conducted for 60 minutes, 5 times each week. Fourteen of 17 patients (82.4%) healed in the TOT group, compared with 5 of 11 (45.5%) in the alginate group ($P = .04$). Median time to closure was also improved by TOT (56 vs 93 days, respectively). The results were particularly impressive considering that the wounds in the TOT group were significantly larger (mean 4.1 vs 1.4 cm^2; $P = .02$) and of greater duration (6.1 vs 3.2 months, $P = $ NS). Although subject to all the flaws inherent in a nonrandomized and nonblinded trial, these results are provocative.

TOT Versus Standard Wound Care

Heng and colleagues[25] reported a prospective study comparing TOT and standard care (wet-to-dry or hydrocolloid dressings) in the care of wounds of various causes, including 39 diabetic foot ulcers and 40 wounds of other types (mostly pressure ulcers). Many patients suffered significant comorbidities. The TOT was delivered at 1.03 atm, 4 h/d, 4 d/wk up to 4 weeks. Complete wound healing was noted in 90% of the TOT group versus 22% of controls. Four of 7 stage IV wounds healed with TOT versus none of 5 in long-term follow-up. The methodology used clouds the results: many patients were not randomized and most patients had more than 1 study wound, making the statistical analysis and interpretation of the data difficult. Wound biopsies were conducted and showed substantial increase in the density of blood vessels and collagen in the TOT wounds. Although acknowledging the limitations of this report, the results argue in favor of TOT compared with standard wound care alone.

Tawfick and Sultan[65] published a nonrandomized comparison of venous leg ulcers treated with TOT and others who were managed using standard therapy (n = 83). At 12 weeks, 80% of patients receiving TOT were healed (median 45 days) compared with 35% of controls (median 182 days; $P<.0001$ for both incidence of healing and time to healing). Patients were allowed to choose whether to be treated with TOT or standard of care. TOT was given in an inpatient setting, with 3-hour treatments twice daily, O_2 at 10 L/min with continuous humidification. Patients were treated until full healing or 12 weeks, whichever came first. Standard of care consisted of wound cleaning, debridement, and Profore (Smith and Nephew, London, United Kingdom) compression dressings 1 to 3 times weekly. Initial patient and wound characteristics were not significantly different between the 2 groups. All wounds were at least 2 years old, and most were larger than 10 cm^2. The methodology raised the question of whether the therapeutic effect came more from mandatory leg elevation 6 hours per day, or from TOT. In 32 of 46 TOT-treated ulcers, granulation tissue developed first in the center of the wound, and then extended peripherally to cover the surface of the lesion.

Clinical Evidence for TOT

Although there is sufficient penetration of TOT to achieve meaningful physiologic effects within the wound bed, the current clinical evidence in favor of this modality needs to be supplemented with more rigorous investigations. In choosing between HBOT and TOT, the benefits for TOT of lower cost and avoidance of potential complications are outweighed by the less potent clinical effect achieved with this approach. Particularly in the case of diabetic foot and leg ulceration, in which there is substantial risk of amputation, the preponderance of data seems to support HBOT in preference to TOT.

HOW MUCH OXYGEN IS OPTIMAL?

Given that correction of wound hypoxia is beneficial to many aspects of healing, it does not necessarily follow that more is better, or that hyperoxygenation of normally nourished wounds confers enough benefit to justify the risks. It is possible that, for some individuals, imposing oxidative stress and excessive ROS may be more harmful than helpful.[2,12] The rate of production of toxic radicals is directly proportional to local oxygen tension.[4] Heng and colleagues[25] make important points about potential negative influences of excess oxygen on wound repair. Unphysiologically high levels of oxygen can react with NADP and be metabolized to ROS in the cytoplasm without the usual catalysis by the mitochondrial cytochrome system, which ordinarily also controls the release of ROS. In this event, the ROS created may be injurious to the host cell (fibroblast, endothelium) rather than serving a useful role in killing foreign organisms. This may be one mechanism by which oxygen exerts brain toxicity, occasionally causing seizures in patients under HBOT.[66] In addition, bypassing the cytochrome system sacrifices production of ATP, so the extra oxygen is wasted. There is the potential for cell cycle arrest and genotoxicity from exposure of cells to pure oxygen.[10,67] Cellular senescence is accelerated in hyperoxic conditions.[12]

Cellular Adaptation to Ambient Oxygen Level

Cells seem to accustom themselves to chronic hypoxia or hyperoxia. For example, the PHD family of proteins, which are known to suppress cellular proliferation, modulate the cell cycle and encourage apoptosis, is expressed when hypoxia is sensed.[68] Cells cultured under 20% oxygen and then subjected to a 5% oxygen environment synthesize higher levels of PHDs; over longer periods of time, PHDs return to baseline levels. Similarly, cells accustomed to culture under 30% oxygen overexpress PHDs when suddenly put under 20% oxygen.[12] Thus there is a hypoxia set point that is tunable. In theory, the optimal oxygen treatment strategy may be to restore hypoxic areas of the wound bed to normal oxygen tension without overtreating and risking oxidative stress.

Individualized Oxygen Dosing

In common practice, nearly all patients receiving HBOT are dosed similarly: 90-minute sessions, once daily at 2.0 to 2.5 ATA. It is possible that this one-size-fits-all approach to dosing might not be appropriate for all patients; some wounds are more hypoxic than others, therefore some may be overdosed and others underdosed. Everyone has endogenous genes that encode antioxidant molecules to protect them against oxidative stress; however, individuals may vary in the levels of expression of these genes and therefore some patients may be less capable than others of dealing with the oxygen load. Real-time wound Po_2 mapping assist understand of the degree of hypoxia in each wound, and could be the basis for more individualized therapy.

REFERENCES

1. Hunt TK. Oxygen and skin wound healing. In: Rovee DT, Maibach HI, editors. The epidermis in wound healing. Boca Raton (FL): CRC Press; 2004. p. 183–97.
2. Chambers AC, Leaper DJ. Role of oxygen in wound healing: a review of evidence. J Wound Care 2011; 20(4):160–4.
3. Ruangsetakit C, Chinsakchai K, Mahawongkajit P, et al. Transcutaneous oxygen tension: a useful predictor of ulcer healing in critical limb ischemia. J Wound Care 2010;19:202–6.
4. Tandara AA, Mustoe TA. Oxygen in wound healing—more than a nutrient. World J Surg 2004;28: 294–300.
5. Scheffield PJ. Tissue oxygen measurements. In: Davis JC, Hunt TK, editors. Problem wounds: the role of oxygen. New York: Elsevier; 1988. p. 17–52.
6. Mustoe TA, O'Shaughnessy K, Kloeters O. Chronic wound pathogenesis and current treatment strategies: a unifying hypothesis. Plast Reconstr Surg 2006;117:S35–41.

7. Schreml S, Szeimies RM, Prantl L, et al. Oxygen in acute and chronic wound healing. Br J Dermatol 2010;163:257–68.

8. Peirce SM, Skalak TC, Rodeheaver GT. Ischemia-reperfusion injury in chronic pressure ulcer formation: a skin model in the rat. Wound Repair Regen 2000;8:68–76.

9. Reid RR, Sull AC, Mogford JE, et al. A novel murine model of cyclical cutaneous ischemia-reperfusion injury. J Surg Res 2004;116:172–80.

10. Gordillo GM, Sen CK. Revisiting the essential role of oxygen in wound healing. Excerpta Med 2003;186:259–63.

11. Ogrin R, Woodward M, Sussman G, et al. Oxygen tension assessment: an overlooked tool for prediction of delayed healing in a clinical setting. Int Wound J 2011;8:435–45.

12. Sen CK. Wound healing essentials: let there be oxygen. Wound Repair Regen 2009;17:1–18.

13. Schreml S, Meier RJ, Wolfbeis OS, et al. 2D luminescence imaging of physiological wound oxygenation. Exp Dermatol 2011;20:550–4.

14. Thackham JA, McElawin DL, Long RJ. The use of hyperbaric oxygen therapy to treat chronic wounds: a review. Wound Repair Regen 2008;16:321–30.

15. Hopf HW, Gibson JJ, Angeles AP, et al. Hyperoxia and angiogenesis. Wound Repair Regen 2005;13:558–64.

16. Siddiqui A, Galiano RD, Connors D, et al. Differential effects of oxygen on human dermal fibroblasts: acute versus chronic hypoxia. Wound Repair Regen 1996;4:211–8.

17. Sashwati R, Khanna S, Alice A, et al. Oxygen sensing by primary cardiac fibroblasts. Circ Res 2003;92:264–71.

18. Mogford JE, Tawil N, Chen A, et al. Effect of age and hypoxia on TGFbeta1 receptor expression and signal transduction in human dermal fibroblasts: impact on cell migration. J Cell Physiol 2002;190:259–65.

19. O'Toole EA, Marinkovich MP, Peavey CL, et al. Hypoxia increases human keratinocyte motility on connective tissue. J Clin Invest 1997;100:2881–91.

20. Mendez MV, Stanley A, Park HY, et al. Fibroblasts cultured from venous ulcers display cellular characteristics of senescence. J Vasc Surg 1998;28:876–83.

21. Schwentker A, Vodovotz Y, Weller R, et al. Nitric oxide and wound repair: role of cytokines? Nitric Oxide 2002;7:1–10.

22. Hehenberger K, Brismar K, Lind F, et al. Dose-dependent hyperbaric oxygen stimulation of human fibroblast proliferation. Wound Repair Regen 1997;5:147–50.

23. Allen D, Maguire J, Mahdavian M, et al. Wound hypoxia and acidosis limit neutrophil bacterial killing mechanisms. Arch Surg 1997;132:991–6.

24. Sen CK. The general case for redox control of wound repair. Wound Repair Regen 2003;11:431–8.

25. Heng MC, Harker J, Csathy G, et al. Angiogenesis in necrotic ulcers treated with hyperbaric oxygen. Ostomy Wound Mgmt 2000;46:18–32.

26. Doctor N, Pandya S, Supe A. Hyperbaric oxygen therapy in diabetic foot. J Postgrad Med 1992;38:112–4.

27. Chylack LT Jr, Brown NP, Bron A, et al. The Roche European American Cataract Trial (REACT): a randomized clinical trial to investigate the efficacy of an oral antioxidant micronutrient mixture to slow progression of age-related cataract. Ophthalmic Epidemiol 2002;9:49–80.

28. Greenberg ER, Baron JA, Tosteson TD, et al. A clinical trial of antioxidant vitamins to prevent colorectal adenoma. Polyp Prevention Study. N Engl J Med 1994;331:141–7.

29. Kaugars GE, Silverman S Jr, Lovas JG, et al. A clinical trial of antioxidant supplements in the treatment of oral leukoplakia. Oral Surg Oral Med Oral Pathol 1994;78:462–8.

30. Ushio-Fukai M, Nakamura Y. Reactive oxygen species and angiogenesis: NADPH oxidase as target for cancer therapy. Cancer Lett 2008;266:37–52.

31. Soberman RJ. Series introduction: the expanding network of redox signaling: new observations, complexities, and perspectives. J Clin Invest 2003;111:571–4.

32. Sen CK, Khanna S, Babior BM, et al. Oxidant-induced vascular endothelial growth factor expression in human keratinocytes and cutaneous wound healing. J Biol Chem 2002;277:33284–90.

33. Roy S, Khanna S, Nallu K, et al. Dermal wound healing is subject to redox control. Mol Ther 2006;13:211–20.

34. Fife CE, Buyukcakir C, Otto GH, et al. The predictive value of transcutaneous oxygen tension measurement in diabetic lower extremity ulcers treated with hyperbaric oxygen therapy: a retrospective analysis of 1,144 patients. Wound Repair Regen 2002;10:198–207.

35. Fries RB, Wallace WA, Roy S. Dermal excisional wound healing in pigs following treatment with topically applied pure oxygen. Mutat Res 2005;579:172–81.

36. Sander AL, Henrich D, Muth CM, et al. In vivo effect of hyperbaric oxygen on wound angiogenesis and epithelialization. Wound Repair Regen 2009;17:179–84.

37. Knighton DR, Halliday B, Hunt TK. Oxygen as an antibiotic. The effect of inspired oxygen on infection. Arch Surg 1984;119:199–204.

38. Hopf HW, Hunt TK, West JM, et al. Wound tissue oxygen tension predicts the risk of wound infection in surgical patients. Arch Surg 1997;132:997–1004.

39. Greif R, Akca O, Horn EP, et al. Supplemental perioperative oxygen to reduce the incidence of surgical-wound infection. N Engl J Med 2000;342:161–7.

40. Belda FJ, Aguillera L, Garcia de la Scuncion J, et al. Supplemental perioperative oxygen and the risk of surgical wound infection: a randomized controlled trial. JAMA 2005;294:2035–42.

41. Chura JC, Boyd A, Argenta PA. Surgical site infections and supplemental perioperative oxygen in colorectal surgery patients: a systematic review. Surg Infect 2007;8:455–61.

42. Meyhoff CS, Wetterslev J, Jorgensen LN, et al. Effect of high perioperative oxygen fraction on surgical site infection and pulmonary complications after abdominal surgery: the PROXI randomized clinical trial. JAMA 2009;302:1543–50.

43. National Collaborating Center for Women's and Children's Health. Surgical site infection. London: RCOG Press; 2008. p. 12.

44. Niinikoski JHA. Clinical hyperbaric oxygen therapy, wound perfusion and transcutaneous oximetry. World J Surg 2004;28:307–11.

45. Boerema I, Meyne NG, Brummelkamp WK, et al. Life without blood. A study of the influence of high atmospheric pressure and hypothermia on dilution of the blood. J Cardiovasc Surg 1960;1:133–46.

46. Kindwall E. A history of hyperbaric medicine. In: Kindwall EP, Whelan HT, editors. Hyperbaric medicine practice. Flagstaff (AZ): Best Publishing Company; 2004. p. 1–20.

47. Barnes RC. Point: hyperbaric oxygen is beneficial for diabetic foot wounds. Clin Infect Dis 2006;43:188–92.

48. Roy S, Khanna S, Bickerstaff AA, et al. Oxygen sensing by primary cardiac fibroblasts: a key role of p21 (Waf1/Cip1/Sdi1). Circ Res 2003;92:264–71.

49. Boykin JV Jr, Baylis C. Hyperbaric oxygen therapy mediates increased nitric oxide production associated with wound healing: a preliminary study. Adv Skin Wound Care 2007;20:382–8.

50. Gallagher KA, Goldstein LJ, Thom SR, et al. Hyperbaric oxygen and bone marrow-derived endothelial progenitor cells in diabetic wound healing. Vascular 2006;14:328–37.

51. Gallagher KA, Liu ZJ, Xiao M, et al. Diabetic impairments in NO-mediated endothelial progenitor cell mobilization and homing are reversed by hyperoxia and SCF-1 alpha. J Clin Invest 2007;117:1249–59.

52. Goldstein LJ, Gallagher KA, Bauer SM, et al. Endothelial progenitor cell release into circulation is triggered by hyperoxia-induced increases in bone marrow nitric oxide. Stem Cells 2006;24:2309–18.

53. Zhao LL, Davidson JD, Wee SC, et al. Effect of hyperbaric oxygen and growth factors on rabbit ear ischemic ulcers. Arch Surg 1994;129:1043–9.

54. Siddiqui A, Davidson JD, Mustoe TA. Ischemic tissue oxygen capacitance after hyperbaric oxygen therapy: a new physiological concept. Plast Reconstr Surg 1997;99:148–55.

55. Roeckl-Wiedmann I, Bennett M, Kranke P. Systematic review of hyperbaric oxygen in the management of chronic wounds. Br J Surg 2005;92:24–32.

56. Kessler L, Bilbault P, Ortega F, et al. Hyperbaric oxygenation accelerates the healing rate of nonischemic chronic diabetic foot ulcers: a prospective randomized study. Diabetes Care 2003;26:2378–82.

57. Faglia E, Favales F, Aldeghi A, et al. Adjunctive systemic hyperbaric oxygen therapy in treatment of severe prevalently ischemic diabetic foot ulcer. A randomized study. Diabetes Care 1996;19:1338–43.

58. Baroni G, Porro T, Faglio E, et al. Hyperbaric oxygen in diabetic gangrene treatment. Diabetes Care 1987;10:81–6.

59. Abidia A, Laden G, Kuhan G, et al. The role of hyperbaric oxygen therapy in ischaemic diabetic lower extremity ulcers: a double-blind randomized-controlled trial. Eur J Vasc Endovasc Surg 2003;25:513–8.

60. Kranke P, Bennett MH, Debus SE, et al. Hyperbaric oxygen therapy for chronic wounds. Cochrane Database Syst Rev 2009;(3). 1–37.

61. Lin TF, Chen SB, Niu KC. The vascular effects of hyperbaric oxygen therapy in treatment of early diabetic foot. Undersea Hyperb Med 2001;28(Suppl):63.

62. Asmis R, Qiao M, Zhao Q. Low flow oxygenation of full-excisional skin wounds on diabetic mice improves wound healing by accelerating wound closure and re-epithelialization. Int Wound J 2010;7:349–57.

63. Gordillo GM, Roy S, Khanna S, et al. Topical oxygen therapy induces vascular endothelial growth factor expression and improves closure of clinically presented chronic wounds. Clin Exp Pharmacol Physiol 2008;35:957–64.

64. Blackman E, Moore C, Hyatt J, et al. Topical wound oxygen therapy in the treatment of severe diabetic foot ulcers: a prospective controlled therapy. Ostomy Wound Mgmt 2010;56:24–31.

65. Tawfick W, Sultan S. Does topical wound oxygen (TWO2) offer an improved outcome over conventional compression dressings (CCD) in the management of refractory venous ulcers (RVU)? A parallel observational comparative study. Eur J Vasc Endovasc Surg 2009;38:125–32.

66. Torbati D, Church DF, Keller JM, et al. Free radical generation in the brain precedes hyperbaric oxygen-induced convulsions. Free Radic Biol Med 1992;13:101–6.

67. Gericke GS. Reactive oxygen species and related haem pathway components as possible epigenetic modifiers in neurobehavioural pathology. Med Hypotheses 2006;66:92–9.

68. Gong W, Suzuki K, Russell M, et al. Function of the ING family of PHD proteins in cancer. Int J Biochem Cell Biol 2005;37:1054–65.

Negative Pressure Wound Therapy: An Algorithm

Kunj K. Desai, MD[a], Edward Hahn, MD[a],
Benson Pulikkotill, MD[a], Edward Lee, MD[b],*

KEYWORDS

- Complications • Clinical evidence • Negative pressure wound therapy • NPWT
- Subatmospheric pressure • Wound healing

KEY POINTS

- Evidence shows negative pressure wound therapy (NPWT) to be effective in reducing wound exudates and increasing granulation tissue formation.
- NPWT derives its beneficial effects on wound healing from multiple interactions with changes effected both on a microscopic as well as a macroscopic level.
- NPWT has specifically proved to be an effective modality for wound therapy in several areas, most notably diabetic foot ulcers, open fractures, mediastinal wounds, and skin grafts.
- The benefits of NPWT are based on principles relevant to wound care and healing in general; NPWT does not ameliorate deleterious effects of local infection, hypoxia, trauma, foreign bodies, or systemic problems such as diabetes, malnutrition, or immunodeficiency, which are most frequently responsible for wound healing delay and chronic wound formation.

INTRODUCTION

The concept of treating wounds with negative or subatmospheric pressure was first described by Fleishmann (**Tables 1–6**).[1] At that time, the wound treatment modality consisted of applying a negative pressure wound dressing consisting of a semiocclusive dressing and a suction device over an open fracture. Negative pressure wound therapy (NPWT) on open fractures resulted in improved granulation tissue formation. Fleishmann and colleagues[2–5] subsequent work described the usefulness in traumatic, acute, and chronic wounds.

Argenta and Morykwas[6] and Morykwas and colleagues[7] reported findings from animal as well as human clinical trials showing the usefulness of NPWT on 300 acute, subacute, and chronic wounds, including a 4-fold increase in blood flow

levels when 125 mm Hg subatmospheric pressure was applied. A significantly increased rate of granulation tissue formation ($P \leq .05$) was reported with continuous (63.3% ± 26.1%) and intermittent (103% ± 35.3%) application of NPWT and tissue bacterial counts were also significantly decreased ($P \leq .05$) after 4 days of application.

Since that time, NPWT has overwhelmed the wound-healing world. The use of subatmospheric pressure on wounds has increased exponentially, as has the number of capable devices available. NPWT can be and has been applied to nearly every region of the body: scalp, face, trunk, and extremities. Certain types of wounds such as open sternal wounds and diabetic foot ulcers have occurred frequently enough for them to provide a large body of evidence. This evidence varies in quality

[a] Department of Surgery, New Jersey Medical School – UMDNJ, 140 Bergen Street, Suite E1620, Newark, NJ 07103, USA; [b] Division of Plastic Surgery, New Jersey Medical School, University of Medicine and Dentistry of New Jersey, 140 Bergen Street, Suite E1620, Newark, NJ 07103, USA
* Corresponding author.
E-mail address: leee9@umdnj.edu

Clin Plastic Surg 39 (2012) 311–324
doi:10.1016/j.cps.2012.05.002
0094-1298/12/$ – see front matter Published by Elsevier Inc

Table 1
Descriptors of evidence levels

Evidence Level	Description
I	High-quality meta-analysis, systematic reviews of randomized controlled trials (RCTs), high-quality RCTs
II	High-quality systemic reviews of case control or cohort studies, high-quality case control or cohort studies
III	Nonanalytical studies (eg, case reports, case series, or in vivo or in vitro studies)
IV	Expert opinion

from observational case reports and series to randomized controlled trials (RCTs).

We have developed an algorithm after careful evaluation and analysis of the scientific literature supporting the use of these devices.

MECHANISM OF ACTION OF NEGATIVE PRESSURE WOUND HEALING

Since antiquity, wound dressings have been used to facilitate and accelerate wound healing. Two concepts that are critical to dressing selection are:

1. Occlusion
2. Absorption.

Wounds treated with occlusive dressings have been shown to re-epithelialize more quickly than wounds left exposed and allowed to dry.[8] Excessive exudates tend to macerate the skin around

Table 2
Evidence-based recommendations for NPWT in venous ulcers

Author	Year	Evidence Level	Evidentiary Bullet
Vuerstaek et al[19]	2006	I	The use of NPWT reduced skin graft preparation time by 58% and also reduced time to overall complete healing by 35%
Korber et al[20]	2008	II	Skin graft take with NPWT 92% vs skin graft alone 67%

wound edges and also encourage bacterial overgrowth, resulting in impaired wound healing, hence the need for absorptive dressings.[9] NPWT fulfills both these basic tenets and provides additional benefits to the healing wound.

NPWT derives its beneficial effects on wound healing from multiple interactions, with changes effected both on a microscopic as well as a macroscopic level.

Tissue Strain

One theory suggests that the subatmospheric pressure induces microdeformations or strain on tissue of between 5% and 20%. This level of strain has been shown to promote cellular proliferation and division, elaboration of growth factors, and angiogenesis.[10] Tissue expansion to expand soft tissue and Ilizarovian distraction osteogenesis to lengthen bones use the same principles of strain.[11,12]

Inflammation Reduction

Second, inflammation generally leads to increased capillary permeability that causes an increase in interstitial fluid: edema. Edema inhibits wound healing by decreasing oxygen and nutrient transport across tissue. Edema also increases the distance between capillaries and healing cells, thereby increasing the likelihood of tissue necrosis. NPWT actively reduces the amount of edema fluid, proteolytic enzymes, acute phase proteins, metalloproteases, proinflammatory mediators and cytokines and increases the blood flow in tissue.[7]

Bacterial Load Reduction

Wounds are often further complicated by bacterial overgrowth and infection, leading to further tissue necrosis and cell death. Infection has also been shown to prolong the inflammatory phase of wound healing, thereby delaying wound repair. The effect of NPWT on infection has been shown by the ability to reduce bacterial load in a wound, decrease interstitial fluid, and improve local blood flow, the combined effect of which is an improvement in the rate at which wound healing occurs.

NPWT ALGORITHM

NPWT has become a mainstay of treatment of acute and chronic wounds. The evidence for use of NPWT is variable. Most clinicians have developed a personal algorithm for application of NPWT, and there have been attempts at creating a consensus statement or guidelines for use of NPWT.[13]

Table 3
Evidence-based recommendations for NPWT in diabetic foot ulcer

Author	Year	Evidence Level	Evidentiary Bullet
McCallon et al[28]	1997	I	The use of NPWT decreased wound surface area compared with saline gauze dressing; however, there was no statistical difference in time to complete healing
Blume et al[26]	2008	I	NPWT seems to be as safe as and more efficacious than advanced moisture wound therapy for the treatment of diabetic foot ulcers with regard to the total number of patients with healed ulcers, time to wound closure, and overall incidence of limb amputation
Armstrong and Lavery[27]	2005	I	NPWT seems to lead to a higher proportion of healed wounds, faster healing rates, and potentially fewer reamputations than standard care

Paramount to use of NPWT are:

1. Primary wound assessment
2. Wound bed preparation
3. Optimization of patient comorbidities.

After control of these issues, we assess each wound individually. We base our decision to use NPWT on the wound characteristics, including:

- Presence of necrotic tissue
- Presence of infected tissue
- What is exposed in the wound bed.

Other wounds such as sternal osteomyelitis have been well studied and these are considered separately. Chronic wounds have been well studied in regard to particular comorbidities such as venous stasis ulcers and diabetic foot ulcers. The use of NPWT is controversial for some uses, such as over flaps, and is well documented for others, such as skin grafts.

Technical aspects of application of NPWT have been studied, but no consensus is clear. Technical modifications include the choice of material under a semiocclusive dressing, the type of semiocclusive dressing, a wound/NPWT device interface, the negative pressure, and the type of pressure (continuous or intermittent). Each of these modifications and evidence for it is reviewed.

WOUND ASSESSMENT AND PREPARATION

The benefits of NPWT are based on certain principles that are relevant to wound care and healing in general. Local infection, hypoxia, trauma, foreign bodies, or systemic problems such as diabetes mellitus, malnutrition, or immunodeficiency are most frequently responsible for delay in wound healing and in the formation of chronic wounds. The addition of NPWT does not ameliorate these deleterious effects.

Table 4
Evidence-based recommendations for NPWT in split-thickness skin graft (STSG)

Author	Year	Evidence Level	Evidentiary Bullet
Llanos et al[65]	2006	I	The use of NPWT significantly diminishes the loss of STSG area, as well as shortening the days of hospital stay
Moisidis et al[66]	2004	I	NPWT significantly improved the qualitative appearance of STSGs compared with standard bolster dressings
Vuerstack et al[19]	2006	I	During the wound bed preparation stage, NPWT seems to be superior to conventional wound care techniques
Korber et al[20]	2008	II	NPWT achieves complete healing in 93% of patients with chronic leg ulcer grafts vs 67% with standard therapy

Table 5
Evidence-based recommendations for NPWT in burns

Author	Year	Evidence Level	Evidentiary Bullet
Kamolz et al[81]	2004	II	Patients with partial-thickness or mixed-thickness burn may benefit from NPWT by reducing edema formation and increasing perfusion
Danks[82]	2010	III	Favorable case report of NPWT being used in a large, single, potentially fatal burn in Iraq
Haslik et al[83]	2004	III	The application of NPWT to burns improves edema and microcirculation, potentially preventing progression of the wound
Molnar et al[84]	2005	III	Did not show the prevention of progression of burns with NPWT; however, it did prove the need for further research
Morykwas et al[40]	1999	III	The application of NPWT to partial-thickness burn injuries prevented progression to a deeper injury in an experimental animal model

For NPWT to be beneficial in healing wounds, several conditions must be fulfilled:

- Paramount to wound healing, regardless of device or dressing choice, is the need for accurate diagnosis. Wound care practitioners must make an accurate diagnosis to provide adequate treatment of underlying medical and wound conditions such as diabetes, peripheral vascular disease, or malignancy.
- Wounds should generally be clean of debris and necrotic tissue. Debridement removes devitalized tissue, which can be a source of endotoxins that inhibit fibroblast and keratinocyte migration into the wound.
- Wounds should have an adequate vascular supply. Angioplasty or arterial bypass grafting may be necessary to ensure adequate oxygenation.
- Compressive garments may improve venous stasis or insufficiency.
- Better glycemic control should be instituted. Glycosylation in diabetes mellitus impairs neutrophil and macrophage phagocytosis of bacteria, prolonging the inflammatory phase of wound healing.
- Infection should be controlled either with systemic antibiotics or local debridement or drainage. Cellulitis prolongs the inflammatory phase by maintaining high levels of proinflammatory cytokines and tissue proteases, which degrade granulation tissue and tissue growth factors, and by delaying collagen deposition.
- Optimization of patient comorbidities and the wound bed are essential.

CONTRAINDICATIONS TO NPWT

There are specific contraindications to NPWT. Kinetic Concepts (San Antonio, TX, USA) has listed the following contraindications for its NPWT vacuum-assisted closure (VAC) product[14]:

- Exposed vessels	- Malignancy
- Anastomotic sites	- Untreated osteomyelitis
- Organs	- Nonenteric and unexplored fistulas
- Nerves	- Necrotic tissue

These contraindications are specifically for the VAC, but they can be generalized to all NPWT devices.

Before initiation of NPWT, the wound must be adequately debrided of necrotic tissue. Evidence of wound infection should be treated before initiation of NPWT.

The use of NPWT in areas with exposed vital organs is contraindicated. Several case reports indicate the development of hemorrhage, anastomotic breakdown, and enteric.[15–18]

NPWT should be used cautiously when:

- There is active bleeding
- The patient is on anticoagulants
- There is difficult wound hemostasis
- Placing the dressing beside blood vessels.

Table 6
Evidence-based recommendations for NPWT in sternal wounds

Author	Year	Evidence Level	Evidentiary Bullet
Damiani et al[41]	2011	I	NPWT reduces hospital stay without affecting overall mortality
Doss et al[46]	2002	II	NPWT shortened wound healing and hospital stay in patients with poststernotomy osteomyelitis
Catarino et al[42]	2000	II	The use of negative pressure suction drainage is a valuable adjunct in the early management of poststernotomy mediastinitis
Domkowski et al[43]	2003	II	NPWT is effective after debridement or before placement of a vascularized tissue flap in infected mediastinal wounds
Moidl et al[45]	2006	II	NPWT therapy after poststernotomy mediastinitis significantly reduces morbidity and mortality; it is also cost-effective
Fleck et al[44]	2002	III	NPWT is an effective and safe adjunct to conventional treatment modalities for the therapy for sternal wound infections

Some of these adverse effects may be mitigated by the addition of a wound contact layer, but this is anecdotal.

The presence of inadequately debrided wounds, as stated, prevents the formation of granulation tissue. The presence of untreated osteomyelitis or grossly contaminated tissue within the vicinity of the wound may lead to abscess formation. The presence of necrotic tissue with eschar, in addition to increasing the infection burden, also inhibits the establishment of effective vacuum across the wound and hence is contraindicated.

The presence of malignancy in the wound is also a contraindication for negative pressure therapy because it may, theoretically, lead to cellular proliferation of malignant cells.

NPWT use is contraindicated on fragile skin resulting from age, chronic steroid use, or collagen vascular disorders. The repeated trauma of dressing changes can inflict severe injury to fragile skin, resulting in the development of more chronic wounds.

NPWT FOR VENOUS ULCERS

Venous stasis ulcers develop when the venous outflow from a lower extremity is compromised, resulting in the pooling of blood, leading to edema, necrosis, and eventually, ulcers of the lower extremities. A standard dressing for chronic venous ulcers has been a compression dressing. However, compression dressings are often insufficient in treating these challenging wounds.

NPWT as Adjunct to Skin Graft

There is strong evidence for the success of NPWT as an adjunct with skin grafting in the treatment of chronic venous ulcers. When applied to chronic venous ulcers in preparation for skin graft, NPWT has been shown to decrease wound preparation time by 58%.[16,19] In addition, the duration of overall complete healing of chronic venous ulcers treated with skin grafts is decreased by 35% when NPWT is applied versus the application of hydrocolloid or alginate dressings.[16] The overall split-thickness skin graft (STSG) take rate is increased by 92% with the use of NPWT versus 67% observed in skin-grafted wounds without NPWT.[17,20] In the same study, patients with diabetes and chronic venous ulcers showed 100% STSG take with the use of NPWT versus 50% take with the absence of NPWT.

NPWT as Primary Treatment

The evidence is poor for the use of NPWT as a primary treatment of chronic venous ulcers. The use of NPWT in such a way often results in increased pain and bleeding. NPWT can damage the delicate skin adjacent to a chronic venous ulcer, further limiting the use of NPWT as a primary instrument in the treatment of chronic venous ulcers. Some investigators have reported the beneficial effects of NPWT using gauze rather than foam, resulting in significantly decreased pain.[21]

Author approach to NPWT for venous ulcers

We use NPWT after STSG for venous ulcers but we do not advocate the use of NPWT as the primary treatment of venous leg ulcers.

NPWT FOR DIABETIC FOOT ULCERS

Diabetic foot ulcers are yet another challenging wound for physicians to treat. Neuropathic changes, arthrosclerosis, and foot deformities often lead to ulceration of the lower extremities. According to the National Institute of Diabetes and Digestive and Kidney Diseases, diabetic foot lesions are responsible for more hospitalizations than any other complication of diabetes. Diabetes is the leading cause of nontraumatic lower extremity amputations in the United States, with approximately 5% of diabetics developing foot ulcers each year and 1% requiring amputation.[22]

The chronic nature of these wounds and debilitating secondary amputations that are often sequelae of these chronic wounds implies a substantial need for optimal wound management. Treatment consists of appropriate glycemic control, debridement, revascularization as needed, treatment of infection, and off- loading of the foot. Removal of devitalized tissue followed by NPWT hastens recovery.

Level 1 data suggest that NPWT assists in the acceleration of wound healing. Seven RCTs, of which 2 were high quality, show this to be the case.[23–28] Armstrong and Lavery[27] reported that:

- More patients in the NPWT group healed their wounds (defined as 100% re-epithelialization with no drainage) versus the standard group (56%–39%, $P = .04$, respectively).
- Rate of healing and of granulation tissue formation was faster in the NPWT group.
- They found trends toward fewer second amputations.

Similar findings were also corroborated by Blume and colleagues[26] in their multicenter RCT. These investigators observed that at 9 months 43.2% of patients with NPWT versus 28.9% of patients receiving advanced moist wound therapy experienced complete wound closure. These data are for patients with diabetic foot ulcers not secondary to ischemia. In wounds secondary to ischemia, revascularization remains the appropriate first line of treatment, although this may not always be feasible. Anecdotal evidence does suggest that even in these patients, NPWT may have some usefulness.[19]

Author Approach to NPWT for Diabetic Foot Ulcers

Patient comorbidities, especially among diabetic patients, must be optimized, including glucose control, peripheral vascular disease, and cardiac disease. We use NPWT extensively for diabetic foot ulcers both as a bridge to surgical closure and as a means to facilitate healing by secondary intention.

OPEN FRACTURES

Data regarding the use of NPWT in acute lower extremity wounds are less clear and warrant further investigation. Most reports regarding wounds and NPWT often do not explicitly differentiate between specific lower extremity wounds or even traumatic wounds. As a result, we are forced to extrapolate some conclusions from these reports as well as case series. NPWT has been shown to be useful in obtaining wound closure in various types of traumatic injuries, including[29–32]:

- Ankle
- Calcaneal
- Pilon and tibial plateau fractures
- Soft tissue defects involving exposed bone, tendon, or hardware
- Hematomas.

The usefulness was also shown in the management of lower extremity fasciotomies, which received NPWT followed by closure either by secondary intent or by skin grafting.[2]

Use of NPWT on open fractures has been well documented. NPWT is most often used as bridge therapy to maintain the wound bed before definitive closure. DeFranzo and colleagues[31] reported a case series that observed NPWT applied to decreased edema of open fractures and decreased circumference of the extremity and size of the wound; 95% of wounds were successfully closed.

Author Approach to NPWT for Open Fractures

In lower extremity traumatic wounds, we use NPWT as a bridge to definitive closure by a vascularized flap or skin graft.

NPWT FOR PRESSURE ULCERS

Pressure ulcers are chronic wounds associated with significant morbidity and mortality. The prevalence of pressure sores in hospitalized patients has been reported to be from 14% to 21% over the last decade and the overall annual cost has recently been estimated to be between 5 billion and 8.5 billion dollars.[33]

One prospective study of 18 patients compared NPWT with traditional wet-to-moist dressings; this study reported some benefit in terms of reduction in wound volume/depth, whereas 2 other smaller studies showed no benefit in terms of wound contraction.[34–36] However, there are data to support the concept of NPWT increasing the prevalence of healing of pressure ulcers by secondary intention.[37] This prospective study of NPWT compared with moist-gauze dressings showed no statistically significant difference in time to closure between the 2 treatment groups overall; however, in a subset analysis of pressure ulcers, wounds in the treatment group achieved closure faster than the control group (mean 10 ± 7.11 days for treatment and 27 ± 10.6 days in control group, $P = .05$). Baharestani and colleagues[38] have also shown that the introduction of NPWT (within 30 days) in the course of the treatment of stage III and stage IV pressure ulcers decreased hospital days of admission. Their study showed that for every day that NPWT is delayed, the patient hospital stay increased by 1 day. Other potential benefits of NPWT include ease of use, increased patient comfort, and decreased frequency of dressing changes. Further investigations are needed to report on the cost-effectiveness of NPWT applied to pressure ulcers.

Author Approach to NPWT for Pressure Ulcers

We use NPWT for pressure ulcers after adequate debridement and initiation of appropriate antibiotics if osteomyelitis is present. However, frequent soiling or the loss of adherence of the semiocclusive dressing may preclude the use of NPWT for pressure ulcers.

NPWT FOR BURNS

Progression of burns from partial thickness to full thickness is brought about by decreased blood flow within the zone of stasis caused by edema and the resulting capillary stasis and thrombosis. NPWT may be ideal to induce the physiologic changes necessary for healing to occur and prevent progression; however, the evidence is not conclusive. There is a lack of evidence supporting the use of NPWT for burn wounds. A Cochrane review[39] of RCTs evaluating safety and effectiveness of topical negative pressure for partial thickness burns revealed only 1 trial, with poor methodological quality. Removal of tissue edema helps reduce the systemic response by removing proinflammatory cells and debris limiting the progression to full thickness. This situation has

been shown in a porcine skin model by Morykwas and colleagues.[40] Although there seems to be theoretic use of NPWT as a treatment adjunct to burns, high-quality evidence is lacking.

Author Approach to NPWT for Burns

We do not routinely use NPWT for acute burns.

NPWT FOR STERNAL WOUNDS

Poststernotomy mediastinitis is a dreadful complication after midline sternotomy. Acute and chronic mediastinitis are associated with a high morbidity and mortality. Traditionally, surgical debridement and mediastinal irrigation with antibiotic solution had been the mainstay of mediastinal infections. Myocutaneous flap coverage of the mediastinum after adequate debridement is also, now, routine. NPWT seems to play a significant role in the management of these wounds either as a primary modality of wound healing or as a secondary means by preparing the wound for flap reconstruction.

The supporting data, barring 1 meta-analysis, are derived primarily from observational studies. Damiani and colleagues,[41] in a meta-analysis of recent data comparing NPWT with conventional therapies, reported a significant reduction in length of hospital stay without any overall impact on mortality. Catarino and colleagues[42] showed in a small, retrospective study that significantly more treatment failures occurred with continuous irrigation than with NPWT. Domkowski and colleagues,[43] in an observational study using NPWT as a single-line treatment or as a bridge to tissue flap surgery, showed very low (3.7%) early mortality.

NPWT is also associated with lower rates of recurrent mediastinitis when followed by delayed primary closure or pectoral muscle flaps compared with revision and primary closure[44] as well as lower costs.[45] Doss and colleagues[46] reported faster wound healing and a shorter length of hospital stay and treatment duration when comparing NPWT with conventional wound management in the treatment of poststernotomy osteomyelitis.

In addition, in mediastinal wounds, vessels and organs are often exposed; caution must be exercised in the use of NPWT in these circumstances.

Author Approach to NPWT for Sternal Wounds

In circumstances in which debridement of wounds via NPWT dressing changes is not desired, we recommend the use of a wound contact layer (see later discussion). This strategy avoids granulation tissue ingrowth into the NPWT filler material or sponge, thereby protecting the underlying tissues. We use NPWT with a wound contact layer for sternal wounds.

NPWT FOR OPEN ABDOMEN

The open abdomen is a challenging situation associated with considerable morbidity and mortality.[47] Abdominal compartment syndrome, intra-abdominal hypertension, infections, and necrotizing fasciitis have all led to the increased use of the open abdomen as a treatment modality. The advent of damage-control laparotomies has also increased the incidence of open abdomen in intensive care unit (ICU) scenarios. The concept is based on a 3-step approach to abdominal injury:

1. An exploratory laparotomy is performed to repair major injuries and also to pack areas of bleeding.
2. Next, the patient is then transferred to a surgical ICU setting for stabilization and resuscitation; often the abdomen is left open during this phase.
3. Once stabilized, the patient is returned to the operating room for more definitive repairs of injuries and potential closure of the abdomen. This procedure may require repeated attempts, during which time the abdomen is open.

The challenges of the open abdomen include:

- Management of insensible fluid losses
- Containment of intra-abdominal organs
- Management of visceral edema
- Prevention of fascial retraction
- Preservation of fascial integrity.

Several different techniques are used to temporarily cover the open abdominal wound. Bogota bags, artificial bur devices, zippers, silos, and so forth have all been used for closure, achieving eventual fascial closure rates of 65% to 100%.[48–53] There is also evidence that NPWT facilitates rapid delayed primary fascial closure, with high success rates and low morbidity.[54–58] Miller and colleagues[58] reported a prospective study of 43 patients who received NPWT during the course of their open abdomen management, achieving fascial closure rates of 88%. In patients with large fascial defects not amenable to primary closure, the inclusion of acellular dermal matrix as a fascial bridge along with NPWT has led to successful delayed closure, with low complication rates.[59] The addition of retention sutured sequential fascial closure to VAC may increase abdominal closure rate in patients with severe abdominal sepsis.[60]

Pliakos and colleagues[60] showed abdominal closure time of 8 days versus 12 for the group treated with dynamic retention sutures in addition to NPWT versus NPWT alone. It should be noted that there is increased granulation tissue formation and a reported increased risk of enterocutaneous fistulae formation with the use of NPWT filler placed directly over exposed bowel.[61] The use of wound contact layer (see later discussion) is recommended to mitigate this risk.[62]

Author Approach to NPWT for Open Abdomen

We routinely use NPWT without dynamic retention sutures to manage open abdomen.

Enterocutaneous fistulae also pose a particularly common problem on many general surgery floors. The mortality associated with these lesions ranges from 5% to 20% with additional increased morbidity.[63] NPWT has been reported in a case series of 91 patients to reduce fistula output and even entirely suppress it.[64] Although encouraging, the paucity of data does not allow for recommendations to be made for the use of NPWT outside specialist units for this type of disease.

NPWT FOR GRAFTS

NPWT has been used instead of traditional bolstering methods to provide skin graft fixation. The initial use of NPWT is in wound bed preparation by the reducing wound size as well as improving the amount of granulation tissue available for grafting. Once the graft has been placed, the NPWT dressing distributes negative pressure uniformly over the surface of the fresh graft, immobilizing the graft with less chance of shearing. Shearing forces allow for the formation of fluid collections and seromas, which interrupt the interface between the graft and the prepared vascular bed. The active removal of fluid from the wound bed helps to prevent this situation and also facilitates inosculation and revascularization. Improved qualitative skin graft take and quantitative improvements in skin graft success (ie, fewer repeat grafts) have been described in observational studies and 2 randomized trials.

In one of the trials, 60 patients were randomly assigned to NPWT dressing connected to an aspiration system versus NPWT dressing not connected to an aspiration system after STSG. NPWT was associated with significant reduction in:

- Loss of graft area: zero versus 4.5 cm^2 in the control group
- Median duration of hospitalization: 13.5 versus 17 days.

Moisidis and colleagues[65] compared a standard bolster dressing with an NPWT dressing, although quantitative graft take was similar between the 2 groups, NPWT significantly improved the qualitative appearance of the graft (epithelialization rates and skin grafts were better than those of the control group in 75% and 85% of cases, respectively).[65,66]

Author Approach to NPWT for Grafts

We routinely use NPWT with a foam sponge and a wound contact layer (Xeroform, Covidien, Mansfield, MA, USA) to help bolster our skin grafts and other grafts.

NPWT FOR FLAPS

The usefulness of NPWT over vascularized flaps is controversial. NPWT has been shown to reduce cutaneous blood flow in healthy individuals, and this effect is more pronounced at extreme negative pressures.[67–69] This reduction in blood flow because of pressure would be a contraindication for its use over a recently created flap.

Morgan and colleagues[70] also reported the loss of 2 flaps, which were ascribed to the pressure intensity. However, NPWT has also been shown to reduce tissue edema and improve venous congestion and contouring of flaps, all of which are considered beneficial.[71–73]

Eisenhardt and colleagues,[74] specifically, reported that NPWT does not increase the risk of flap failure rates or complications. In their study of 26 patients undergoing microsurgical reconstruction of posttraumatic lower extremity soft tissue defects using NPWT, only 2 flap failures were observed (in patients with peripheral vascular disease). Furthermore, NPWT also reduces the inflammatory response seen in free muscle flaps as a result of ischemia/reperfusion injury as well as providing a protective effect by reducing muscle tissue apoptosis and damage.[72] Further evidence supporting the use of NPWT over flaps is necessary before definitive recommendations can be made.

Author Approach to NPWT for Flaps

We routinely treat pedicled myofascial flaps with NPWT to bolster skin grafts. We do not use NPWT on cutaneous flaps.

NPWT INTRINSIC VARIABLES

After determining that NPWT would be beneficial for a particular wound, we assess several other variables intrinsic to the application of NPWT. NPWT application variables include type of filler material, wound contact layer, and pressure level.

Filler Material

The material used under the occlusive dressing may include black foam (polyurethane), white foam (polyvinyl alcohol [Kinetic Concepts]), or gauze. These materials have proved to be nearly equivalent in transmitting pressure and removal of wound exudates. Clinically, foam and gauze have had similar results in terms of development of granulation tissue and wound contraction; however, foam does result in more wound contraction in larger wounds.[21,75] The black foam is most often used for convenience. Based on anecdotal evidence, in deep wounds with a small surface opening or complex internal geometry, gauze may be preferable to avoid possible retention of foam within the wound. For skin grafts, black foam is routinely used with a wound contact layer and results in an increased percentage of graft take.[20,65] Although no strong evidence exists advocating for the use of 1 type of filler material over the other to accelerate wound healing, there are level 1 data to support the use of gauze to decrease pain associated with dressing changes.[21] This situation is believed to be caused by the lesser degree of tissue ingrowth into the gauze.

Wound Contact Layer

A wound contact layer has been defined as a thin layer of material between the wound bed and the NPWT filler material. A wound contact layer should ideally allow the transmission of the negative pressure across it, allowing fluid egress as well as preventing the wound bed from becoming adherent to the filler material secondary to tissue ingrowth. This strategy allows for easier removal of the filler material, leading to less damage to underlying structures during dressing changes. The wound contact layer also makes the removal of filler material less painful for patients. We routinely use a wound contact layer in mediastinal wounds. We routinely use Xeroform as a wound contact layer when using NPWT to help skin graft adherence. There are concerns that the wound contact layer may decrease fluid egress from the wound bed or affect the transference of pressure to the wound bed.[76] The use of a wound contact layer is recommended when NPWT is to be applied on exposed bowel or mediastinal wounds.

NPWT Pressure Level

The choice of pressure level for NPWT is 2-fold:

1. The decision as to what pressure would be optimal for the wound
2. The decision as to whether the pressure should be continuous or intermittent.

The commonly accepted pressure of 125 mm Hg was suggested after studying wound granulation at pressures of 25 mm Hg, 125 mm Hg, and 500 mm Hg. Wounds treated at 25 mm Hg failed to show granulation, and those treated at 500 mm Hg had malformations of granulation tissue.[77] Wounds treated at 125 mm Hg had formation of granulation tissue, but this pressure was not further compared with 75 mm Hg, 200 mm Hg, or other closer pressures to better determine the optimal pressure.

For some patients, there seems to be a correlation between increasing negative pressure and pain.[68]

The alternating of pressure from 0 mm Hg to 125 mm Hg is believed to accelerate the formation of granulation tissue by increasing the frequency and intensity of macrodeformations across the wound bed. However, in practice, the use of alternating pressure has been difficult. Patients may experience pain from the continuous contraction and relaxation. The wound may accumulate moisture during the off cycle. These wound exudates often leak underneath the occlusive dressing, leading to loss of adherence and subsequent loss of pressure. A possible method of obviating these issues is by cycling between a low and a high pressure setting that maintains a constant negative pressure yet still achieves the desired intermittence.

We consistently use NPWT at 125 mm Hg on a continuous cycle. The pressure can be reduced to 75 mm Hg for patients who experience pain with application of NPWT.

COMPLICATIONS OF NPWT

Twelve deaths and 174 injuries associated with NPWT systems have been reported to the US Food and Drug Administration since 2007.[78]

Infection

Wound infections occurred in more than half of these cases, most of which were related to the retention of dressing pieces in the wounds. These patients experienced delayed recovery and required wound exploration, surgical removal of dead tissue (wound debridement), and drainage.

Bleeding

Bleeding continues to be the cause of the most serious adverse events, and was reported in 89 patients, including 9 death reports. Bleeding occurred in patients who had blood vessel grafts, wound infections, those receiving medicine for blood clots, and during removal of dressings attached to the tissues. Bleeding contributed to shock, low blood pressure, and swelling containing blood (hematoma). Some of the patients who experienced bleeding required additional surgery to stop the bleeding, blood transfusions, admission to the emergency room, and hospitalization.

Demographics

Most of the death and injury reports indicated that the patients were receiving NPWT at home or in a nursing home or long-term care facility.

Avoidance

Avoidance of these complications can be difficult. We carefully select patients for NPWT and ensure that all patients are either transferred to a facility familiar with the device or to a home nursing service with the device.

SOCIOECONOMIC IMPACT OF NPWT

In terms of the cost of treatment, NPWT is associated with a higher initial cost of materials compared with traditional dressings, yet it is still cost-effective overall.[79] Philbeck and colleagues, in a retrospective analysis of healing rates, reported that an average 22.2 cm^2 wound would take 97 days to heal at a cost of $14,546 with NPWT versus 247 days and $23,465 for wounds treated with traditional therapy. Braakenburg and colleagues[80] also reported the usefulness of NPWT in improving outcomes and reducing the use of nursing resources. This finding, along with the decrease in dressing changes, results in improved patient satisfaction.

SUMMARY

NPWT has become a major component of wound care therapy and has been shown to be effective in the treatment of acute and chronic wounds. Whether used as an end therapy or a bridge to surgery, evidence shows NPWT to be effective in reducing wound exudates and increasing granulation tissue formation. NPWT has specifically proved to be an effective modality for wound therapy in several areas, most notably diabetic foot ulcers, open fractures, mediastinal wounds, and skin grafts. However, in our experience, the use of NPWT on venous stasis ulcers and burns in particular has been less than satisfactory.

Our algorithm stresses individualized evaluation and treatment of each wound and patient. Additional research will help to create better, substantiated guidelines.

REFERENCES

1. Fleischmann W, Strecker W, Bombelli M, et al. Vacuum sealing as treatment of soft tissue damage in open fractures. Unfallchirurg 1993;96(9):488–92 [in German].
2. Fleischmann W, Lang E, Kinzl L. Vacuum assisted wound closure after dermatofasciotomy of the lower extremity. Unfallchirurg 1996;99(4):283–7 [in German].
3. Fleischmann W, Russ M, Marquardt C. Closure of defect wounds by combined vacuum sealing with instrumental skin expansion. Unfallchirurg 1996; 99(12):970–4 [in German].
4. Fleischmann W, Lang E, Russ M. Treatment of infection by vacuum sealing. Unfallchirurg 1997;100(4): 301–4 [in German].
5. Thoner B, Fleischmann W, Moch D. Wound treatment by vacuum sealing. Krankenpfl J 1998;36(3): 78–82 [in German].
6. Argenta LC, Morykwas MJ. Vacuum-assisted closure: a new method for wound control and treatment: clinical experience. Ann Plast Surg 1997;38(6):563–76 [discussion: 577].
7. Morykwas MJ, Argenta LC, Shelton-Brown EI, et al. Vacuum-assisted closure: a new method for wound control and treatment: animal studies and basic foundation. Ann Plast Surg 1997;38(6):553–62.
8. Winter GD. Formation of the scab and the rate of epithelization of superficial wounds in the skin of the young domestic pig. Nature 1962;193: 293–4.
9. Bishop SM, Walker M, Rogers AA, et al. Importance of moisture balance at the wound-dressing interface. J Wound Care 2003;12(4):125–8.
10. Saxena V, Hwang CW, Huang S, et al. Vacuum-assisted closure: microdeformations of wounds and cell proliferation. Plast Reconstr Surg 2004;114(5): 1086–96 [discussion: 1097–8].
11. Ilizarov GA. The tension-stress effect on the genesis and growth of tissues: Part II. The influence of the rate and frequency of distraction. Clin Orthop Relat Res 1989;(239):263–85.
12. Ilizarov GA. The tension-stress effect on the genesis and growth of tissues. Part I. The influence of stability of fixation and soft-tissue preservation. Clin Orthop Relat Res 1989;(238):249–81.
13. Birke-Sorensen H, Malmsjo M, Rome P, et al. Evidence-based recommendations for negative pressure wound therapy: treatment variables (pressure levels, wound filler and contact layer)–steps towards an international consensus. J Plast Reconstr Aesthet Surg 2011;64(Suppl):S1–16.
14. Kinetic Concepts Inc. V.A.C. therapy indications and contraindications. Available at: http://www.kci1.com/KCI1/indicationsandcontraindications. Accessed January 17, 2012.
15. White RA, Miki RA, Kazmier P, et al. Vacuum-assisted closure complicated by erosion and hemorrhage of the anterior tibial artery. J Orthop Trauma 2005; 19(1):56–9.
16. Grauhan O, Navarsadyan A, Hussmann J, et al. Infectious erosion of aorta ascendens during vacuum-assisted therapy of mediastinitis. Interact Cardiovasc Thorac Surg 2010;11(4):493–4.
17. Kiessling AH, Lehmann A, Isgro F, et al. Tremendous bleeding complication after vacuum-assisted sternal closure. J Cardiothorac Surg 2011;6:16.
18. Fischer JE. A cautionary note: the use of vacuum-assisted closure systems in the treatment of gastrointestinal cutaneous fistula may be associated with higher mortality from subsequent fistula development. Am J Surg 2008;196(1):1–2.
19. Vuerstaek JD, Vainas T, Wuite J, et al. State-of-the-art treatment of chronic leg ulcers: a randomized controlled trial comparing vacuum-assisted closure (V.A.C.) with modern wound dressings. J Vasc Surg 2006;44(5):1029–37 [discussion: 1038].
20. Korber A, Franckson T, Grabbe S, et al. Vacuum assisted closure device improves the take of mesh grafts in chronic leg ulcer patients. Dermatology 2008;216(3):250–6.
21. Dorafshar AH, Franczyk M, Gottlieb LJ, et al. A prospective randomized trial comparing subatmospheric wound therapy with a sealed gauze dressing and the standard vacuum-assisted closure device. Ann Plast Surg 2011. [Epub ahead of print].
22. Reiber G, Boyko E, Smith DG. Lower extremity foot ulcers and amputations in diabetes. In: Harris MI, Cowie CC, Stern MP, et al, editors. Diabetes in America. 2nd edition. Washington, DC: U.S. Department of Health and Human Services, Public Health Service, National Institutes of Health; 1995. [Chapter: 18].
23. Sepulveda G, Espindola M, Maureira M, et al. Negative-pressure wound therapy versus standard wound dressing in the treatment of diabetic foot amputation. A randomised controlled trial. Cir Esp 2009;86(3):171–7 [in Spanish].
24. Eginton MT, Brown KR, Seabrook GR, et al. A prospective randomized evaluation of negative-pressure wound dressings for diabetic foot wounds. Ann Vasc Surg 2003;17(6):645–9.
25. Akbari A, Moodi H, Ghiasi F, et al. Effects of vacuum-compression therapy on healing of diabetic foot ulcers: randomized controlled trial. J Rehabil R D 2007;44(5):631–6.
26. Blume PA, Walters J, Payne W, et al. Comparison of negative pressure wound therapy using vacuum-assisted closure with advanced moist wound therapy in the treatment of diabetic foot ulcers: a multicenter randomized controlled trial. Diabetes Care 2008;31(4):631–6.
27. Armstrong DG, Lavery LA. Negative pressure wound therapy after partial diabetic foot amputation:

a multicentre, randomised controlled trial. Lancet 2005;366(9498):1704–10.

28. McCallon SK, Knight CA, Valiulus JP, et al. Vacuum-assisted closure versus saline-moistened gauze in the healing of postoperative diabetic foot wounds. Ostomy Wound Manage 2000;46(8): 28–32, 34.

29. Mullner T, Mrkonjic L, Kwasny O, et al. The use of negative pressure to promote the healing of tissue defects: a clinical trial using the vacuum sealing technique. Br J Plast Surg 1997;50(3):194–9.

30. Greer S, Kasabian A, Thorne C, et al. The use of a subatmospheric pressure dressing to salvage a Gustilo grade IIIB open tibial fracture with concomitant osteomyelitis to avert a free flap. Ann Plast Surg 1998;41(6):687.

31. DeFranzo AJ, Argenta LC, Marks MW, et al. The use of vacuum-assisted closure therapy for the treatment of lower-extremity wounds with exposed bone. Plast Reconstr Surg 2001;108(5):1184–91.

32. Stannard JP, Robinson JT, Anderson ER, et al. Negative pressure wound therapy to treat hematomas and surgical incisions following high-energy trauma. J Trauma 2006;60(6):1301–6.

33. Fogerty MD, Abumrad NN, Nanney L, et al. Risk factors for pressure ulcers in acute care hospitals. Wound Repair Regen 2008;16(1):11–8.

34. Joseph E, Hamori CA, Bergman S, et al. A prospective randomized trial of vacuum assisted closure versus standard therapy of chronic nonhealing wounds. Wounds 2000;12(3):60–7.

35. Ford CN, Reinhard ER, Yeh D, et al. Interim analysis of a prospective, randomized trial of vacuum-assisted closure versus the healthpoint system in the management of pressure ulcers. Ann Plast Surg 2002;49(1):55–61 [discussion: 61].

36. Wanner MB, Schwarzl F, Strub B, et al. Vacuum-assisted wound closure for cheaper and more comfortable healing of pressure sores: a prospective study. Scand J Plast Reconstr Surg Hand Surg 2003;37(1):28–33.

37. Mody GN, Nirmal IA, Duraisamy S, et al. A blinded, prospective, randomized controlled trial of topical negative pressure wound closure in India. Ostomy Wound Manage 2008;54(12):36–46.

38. Baharestani MM, Houliston-Otto DB, Barnes S. Early versus late initiation of negative pressure wound therapy: examining the impact on home care length of stay. Ostomy Wound Manage 2008;54(11):48–53.

39. Molnar JA. Applications of negative pressure wound therapy to thermal injury. Ostomy Wound Manage 2004;50(Suppl 4A):17–9.

40. Morykwas MJ, David LR, Schneider AM, et al. Use of subatmospheric pressure to prevent progression of partial-thickness burns in a swine model. J Burn Care Rehabil 1999;20(1 Pt 1):15–21.

41. Damiani G, Pinnarelli L, Sommella L, et al. Vacuum-assisted closure therapy for patients with infected sternal wounds: a meta-analysis of current evidence. J Plast Reconstr Aesthet Surg 2011; 64(9):1119–23.

42. Catarino PA, Chamberlain MH, Wright NC, et al. High-pressure suction drainage via a polyurethane foam in the management of poststernotomy mediastinitis. Ann Thorac Surg 2000;70(6):1891–5.

43. Domkowski PW, Smith ML, Gonyon DL Jr, et al. Evaluation of vacuum-assisted closure in the treatment of poststernotomy mediastinitis. J Thorac Cardiovasc Surg 2003;126(2):386–90.

44. Fleck TM, Fleck M, Moidl R, et al. The vacuum-assisted closure system for the treatment of deep sternal wound infections after cardiac surgery. Ann Thorac Surg 2002;74(5):1596–600 [discussion: 1600].

45. Moidl R, Fleck T, Giovanoli P, et al. Cost effectiveness of V.A.C. therapy after post-sternotomy mediastinitis. Zentralbl Chir 2006;131(Suppl 1):S189–90.

46. Doss M, Martens S, Wood JP, et al. Vacuum-assisted suction drainage versus conventional treatment in the management of poststernotomy osteomyelitis. Eur J Cardiothorac Surg 2002;22(6):934–8.

47. Barker DE, Kaufman HJ, Smith LA, et al. Vacuum pack technique of temporary abdominal closure: a 7-year experience with 112 patients. J Trauma 2000;48(2):201–6 [discussion: 206–7].

48. Miller PR, Thompson JT, Faler BJ, et al. Late fascial closure in lieu of ventral hernia: the next step in open abdomen management. J Trauma 2002;53(5): 843–9.

49. DeFranzo AJ, Pitzer K, Molnar JA, et al. Vacuum-assisted closure for defects of the abdominal wall. Plast Reconstr Surg 2008;121(3):832–9.

50. Garner GB, Ware DN, Cocanour CS, et al. Vacuum-assisted wound closure provides early fascial reapproximation in trauma patients with open abdomens. Am J Surg 2001;182(6):630–8.

51. Cothren CC, Moore EE, Johnson JL, et al. One hundred percent fascial approximation with sequential abdominal closure of the open abdomen. Am J Surg 2006;192(2):238–42.

52. Diaz JJ Jr, Dutton WD, Ott MM, et al. Eastern Association for the Surgery of Trauma: a review of the management of the open abdomen—part 2 "Management of the open abdomen". J Trauma 2011;71(2):502–12.

53. Koniaris LG, Hendrickson RJ, Drugas G, et al. Dynamic retention: a technique for closure of the complex abdomen in critically ill patients. Arch Surg 2001;136(12):1359–62 [discussion: 1363].

54. Perez D, Wildi S, Clavien PA. The use of an abdominal vacuum-dressing system in the management of abdominal wound complications. Adv Surg 2007;41: 121–31.

55. Perez D, Wildi S, Demartines N, et al. Prospective evaluation of vacuum-assisted closure in abdominal

compartment syndrome and severe abdominal sepsis. J Am Coll Surg 2007;205(4):586–92.

56. Petersson U, Acosta S, Bjorck M. Vacuum-assisted wound closure and mesh-mediated fascial traction–a novel technique for late closure of the open abdomen. World J Surg 2007;31(11):2133–7.

57. Suliburk JW, Ware DN, Balogh Z, et al. Vacuum-assisted wound closure achieves early fascial closure of open abdomens after severe trauma. J Trauma 2003;55(6):1155–60 [discussion: 1160–1].

58. Miller PR, Meredith JW, Johnson JC, et al. Prospective evaluation of vacuum-assisted fascial closure after open abdomen: planned ventral hernia rate is substantially reduced. Ann Surg 2004;239(5):608–14 [discussion: 614–6].

59. de Moya MA, Dunham M, Inaba K, et al. Long-term outcome of acellular dermal matrix when used for large traumatic open abdomen. J Trauma 2008;65(2):349–53.

60. Pliakos I, Papavramidis TS, Mihalopoulos N, et al. Vacuum-assisted closure in severe abdominal sepsis with or without retention sutured sequential fascial closure: a clinical trial. Surgery 2010;148(5):947–53.

61. Rao M, Burke D, Finan PJ, et al. The use of vacuum-assisted closure of abdominal wounds: a word of caution. Colorectal Dis 2007;9(3):266–8.

62. Shaikh IA, Ballard-Wilson A, Yalamarthi S, et al. Use of topical negative pressure in assisted abdominal closure does not lead to high incidence of enteric fistulae. Colorectal Dis 2010;12(9):931–4.

63. Levy E, Frileux P, Cugnenc PH, et al. High-output external fistulae of the small bowel: management with continuous enteral nutrition. Br J Surg 1989;76(7):676–9.

64. Wainstein DE, Fernandez E, Gonzalez D, et al. Treatment of high-output enterocutaneous fistulas with a vacuum-compaction device. A ten-year experience. World J Surg 2008;32(3):430–5.

65. Moisidis E, Heath T, Boorer C, et al. A prospective, blinded, randomized, controlled clinical trial of topical negative pressure use in skin grafting. Plast Reconstr Surg 2004;114(4):917–22.

66. Llanos S, Danilla S, Barraza C, et al. Effectiveness of negative pressure closure in the integration of split thickness skin grafts: a randomized, double-masked, controlled trial. Ann Surg 2006;244(5):700–5.

67. Kairinos N, Voogd AM, Botha PH, et al. Negative-pressure wound therapy II: negative-pressure wound therapy and increased perfusion. Just an illusion? Plast Reconstr Surg 2009;123(2):601–12.

68. Kairinos N, Solomons M, Hudson DA. Negative-pressure wound therapy I: the paradox of negative-pressure wound therapy. Plast Reconstr Surg 2009;123(2):589–98 [discussion: 599–600].

69. Wackenfors A, Gustafsson R, Sjogren J, et al. Blood flow responses in the peristernal thoracic wall during vacuum-assisted closure therapy. Ann Thorac Surg 2005;79(5):1724–30 [discussion: 1730–1].

70. Morgan K, Brantigan CO, Field CJ, et al. Reverse sural artery flap for the reconstruction of chronic lower extremity wounds in high-risk patients. J Foot Ankle Surg 2006;45(6):417–23.

71. Hanasono MM, Skoracki RJ. Securing skin grafts to microvascular free flaps using the vacuum-assisted closure (VAC) device. Ann Plast Surg 2007;58(5):573–6.

72. Eisenhardt SU, Schmidt Y, Thiele JR, et al. Negative pressure wound therapy reduces the ischaemia/reperfusion-associated inflammatory response in free muscle flaps. J Plast Reconstr Aesthet Surg 2012;65(5):640–9.

73. Bannasch H, Iblher N, Penna V, et al. A critical evaluation of the concomitant use of the implantable Doppler probe and the vacuum assisted closure system in free tissue transfer. Microsurgery 2008;28(6):412–6.

74. Eisenhardt SU, Momeni A, Iblher N, et al. The use of the vacuum-assisted closure in microsurgical reconstruction revisited: application in the reconstruction of the posttraumatic lower extremity. J Reconstr Microsurg 2010;26(9):615–22.

75. Malmsjo M, Lindstedt S, Ingemansson R. Effects of foam or gauze on sternum wound contraction, distension and heart and lung damage during negative-pressure wound therapy of porcine sternotomy wounds. Interact Cardiovasc Thorac Surg 2011;12(3):349–54.

76. Jones SM, Banwell PE, Shakespeare PG. Interface dressings influence the delivery of topical negative-pressure therapy. Plast Reconstr Surg 2005;116(4):1023–8.

77. Morykwas MJ, Faler BJ, Pearce DJ, et al. Effects of varying levels of subatmospheric pressure on the rate of granulation tissue formation in experimental wounds in swine. Ann Plast Surg 2001;47(5):547–51.

78. Food and Drug Administration Safety Communication: Update on serious complications associated with negative pressure wound therapy systems. 2011. Available at: http://www.fda.gov/MedicalDevices/Safety/AlertsandNotices/ucm244211.htm. Accessed March 18, 2012.

79. Philbeck TE Jr, Whittington KT, Millsap MH, et al. The clinical and cost effectiveness of externally applied negative pressure wound therapy in the treatment of wounds in home healthcare Medicare patients. Ostomy Wound Manage 1999;45(11):41–50.

80. Braakenburg A, Obdeijn MC, Feitz R, et al. The clinical efficacy and cost effectiveness of the vacuum-assisted closure technique in the management of acute and chronic wounds: a randomized controlled trial. Plast Reconstr Surg 2006;118(2):390–7 [discussion: 398–400].

81. Kamolz LP, Andel H, Haslik W, et al. Use of subatmospheric pressure therapy to prevent burn wound

progression in human: first experiences. Burns 2004;30(3):253–8.

82. Danks RR, Lairet K. Innovations in caring for a large burn in the Iraq war zone. J Burn Care & Res 2010; 31(4):665–9.

83. Haslik W, Kamolz LP, Andel H, et al. The use of subatmospheric pressure to prevent burn wound progression: first experiences in burn wound treatment. Zentralbl Chir 2004;129(Suppl 1):S62–3 [in German].

84. Molnar JA, Simpson JL, Voignier DM, et al. Management of an acute thermal injury with subatmospheric pressure. J Burns Wounds 2005; 4:e5.

Sophisticated Surgical Solutions for Complex Wound Problems

Simon G. Talbot, MD, Julian J. Pribaz, MD*

KEYWORDS

• Wound • Reconstruction • Flap • Microsurgery

KEY POINTS

- Planning is critical to the outcome of all plastic surgery procedures.
- Keep a "lifeboat," as one never knows when a problem will recur or an initial solution will fail.
- Replace "like with like" to ensure an optimal reconstruction using the best available tissue.
- Use all spare parts before taking tissue from a virgin donor site.
- Replant when possible, as amputated parts are still typically the best reconstructive option.
- Preserve length whenever possible in reconstructing extremities to maximize functionality.
- Consider all tissue layers and, where possible, laminate or fold flaps to obtain lining where this is needed.
- Innovate when undertaking complex wound reconstruction as more elegant solutions may be available to those who think laterally.

INTRODUCTION

Plastic surgery has traditionally been thought of as "surgery of the skin and its contents." Because of this breadth and scope, plastic surgeons have been guided by the reconstructive ladder, consisting of a hierarchy of techniques:

- Healing by secondary intention
- Primary closure
- Delayed primary closure
- Split-thickness skin grafting
- Full-thickness skin grafting
- Tissue expansion
- Random flaps
- Axial flaps
- Free flaps.

Each of these options can be used individually, in combination, or with multiple variations. Together they form the complete armamentarium of the plastic surgeon, and allow complex wound problems to be repaired while maintaining optimal form and function.

The advent of microsurgery in the 1970s allowed a quantum leap in terms of reconstructive options.[1,2] Free tissue transfer has allowed coverage of larger and more complicated defects with adequate quantities of tissue, "like-with-like" tissue, and even multiple tissue types in the forms of composite tissue transfers. Tailored flaps are able to be produced using distant tissue that most appropriately replicates lost tissue; this may even take the form of prefabricated or prelaminated flaps where necessary.[3–8] In addition, free tissue transfer has multiplied the options and provided "lifeboats," which may be necessary in complex reconstructions.

Free (and pedicled) tissue transfer has been further augmented by a thorough understanding

Disclosures: The authors have no financial disclosures. This work has not received any research funding.
Division of Plastic Surgery, Department of Surgery, Brigham and Women's Hospital, Boston, 75 Francis Street, Boston, MA 02115, USA
* Corresponding author.
E-mail address: jpribaz@partners.org

Clin Plastic Surg 39 (2012) 325–340
doi:10.1016/j.cps.2012.05.003

of perforator anatomy, which has brought about the use of freestyle flaps.[9] These flaps further expand the options for donor sites while minimizing donor-site morbidity and maximizing the concept of like-with-like tissue transfer.

A further extension of these concepts has occurred over the last decade, during which time there has been a move from reconstruction to restoration.[10] Restoration using tissue transplantation can provide the most perfect match for complex tissue replacement. In this situation plastic surgeons are no longer "making do" with similar tissues, but are truly restoring anatomy. This approach is especially relevant to facial or hand transplantation, where no other part of the body produces an ideal alternative to the original tissue.[11]

Despite the principles of the reconstructive ladder, free tissue transfer, and tissue restoration, and the ever increasing options available to plastic surgeons through innovative use of multiple modalities, there are numerous principles that hold true. These principles underscore some of the more sophisticated surgical solutions for complex wound problems. Each section in this article is dedicated to a principle necessary for complex wound reconstruction.

PLANNING IS CRITICAL

Careful planning of preoperative, operative, and postoperative steps applies to all reconstructive surgery. However, planning is particularly important when undertaking unique or tailor-made reconstructive operations, and critical when reconstruction requires multiple steps. This reasoning is particularly true for complex wound problems whereby many plastic surgical operations are based on principles rather than on repetitive and sequenced operations. In these situations it is very important to ensure maintenance of tissue vascularity and viability while not burning bridges for future options or stages. Expecting the unexpected through careful planning is crucial.

Planning involves several steps. A thorough literature review or discussion with other experts may be important when novel or innovative techniques are being used. This action may necessitate drawing out expected vascular patterns, nerves, and flap dimensions to make sure that a plan is executable. In the operating room, testing the reach of a flap is important to ensure that it is adequate for the intended coverage. In some instances, alginate molds may allow the 3-dimensionality of a reconstruction to be accommodated.[12] During follow-up, photographs of intraoperative and postoperative findings are important in order to learn from a complex reconstruction and its results.

Unique repairs require planning more than any other situation. **Fig. 1** demonstrates a traumatic volar thumb injury. Despite significant soft-tissue defects, maintenance of the thumb is crucial to maintaining hand function. The first stage in this

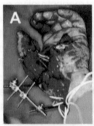
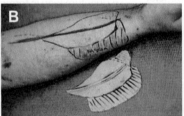
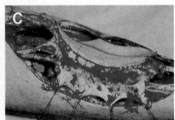
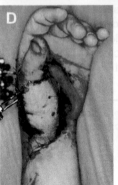
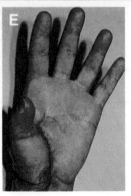

Fig. 1. (*A–E*) Traumatic volar thumb injury treated with a "tailored" radial forearm flap is taken to fit the defect exactly, and the fascia is used to recreate a gliding surface for the reconstructed tendon.

repair involves debridement of all nonviable tissue. An external fixator is placed to maintain a bony stability while the remaining soft tissues are repaired and heal. The flexor pollicis longus tendon is repaired using a tendon graft. A tailored radial forearm flap is then used, and the underlying vascularized fascia maintained with it to allow a gliding surface for the tendons. Through careful planning, a very functional and cosmetically acceptable result is obtained.

KEEP A "LIFEBOAT"

Keeping a lifeboat is another very important principle that underscores complex wound repair. Sophisticated solutions do not always work as planned, and alternatives must always be kept in mind. Experienced plastic surgeons are aware that the part of the flap that fails is typically the most distal aspect, and this is usually the most important part needed to cover critical structures. As a result, anticipating potential complications or

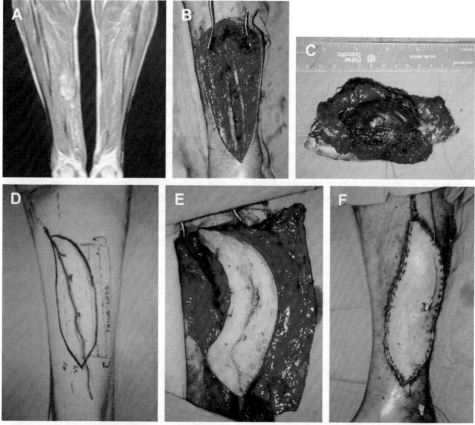

Fig. 2. (A–G) Vascularized fascia may be used to reconstruct an Achilles tendon.

flap losses and maintaining an alternative wherever possible is important. Lifeboat alternatives may be required intraoperatively or for a second procedure, and it is important not to burn bridges in terms of vascularity, scarring, or compromising donor sites unnecessarily.

Where lifeboats are limited, prefabrication of a flap may be used.[3,13] This technique involves bringing a blood supply to tissues where no axial blood supply previously existed. Prefabricating a flap allows donor sites, which could not otherwise be used, to be transferred on their implanted vascular pedicle, after a period (usually 8 weeks) of revascularization.

REPLACE LIKE WITH LIKE

The principle of replacing like tissue with like tissue is central to complex wound reconstruction and continues to be a fundamental principle of plastic surgery. Like tissues may require significant innovation. **Fig. 2** shows an example of Achilles tendon reconstruction after a sarcoma resection. Although native Achilles tendon is unavailable, the use of folded vascularized fascia lata allows a close approximation and allows not only vascularized coverage of the skin defect but also functional reconstruction of the Achilles tendon.

USE ALL SPARE PARTS

Another key principle is to consider the option of using spare parts.[14] Using parts that would otherwise be discarded including amputated parts, "dog ears" at wound edges, or segmentally resected tissue is an ideal way to minimize donor-site morbidity while potentially preserving irreplaceable tissue. The opportunity to replant a part is the ultimate example of replacing like tissue with like tissue.

In any surgery involving complex reconstruction, the surgeon should avoid throwing away any tissue, including fat, skin, and vessels for grafting, until a reconstruction is completely finished, to avoid the need to harvest further tissues later.

The principle of using all spare parts is particularly applicable in the hand. Using tailored grafts and flaps from adjacent fingers or the feet and using tissue rearrangement, heterotopic replantation, or ectopic replantation allows the surgeon to maximize function and minimize donor-site morbidity.[15–17]

One such example of this is the use of a fascial extension and palmaris tendon when using a radial forearm flap to provide a gliding and vascularized graft (**Fig. 3**).

Another example of this principle is shown in **Fig. 4**. The thumb is so valuable that rarely will a reconstruction from scratch be as good as a native thumb. Maintenance of whatever is left after severe trauma is attempted at the primary stage. Additional tissue can then be transferred as a free flap from such sites of the toe, giving an excellent esthetic and functional reconstruction.

Segmental injuries either from trauma or surgical resections can cause the loss of proximal tissue while distal tissue remains viable. When this occurs in the lower extremity, a Van Nes rotationplasty can convert an above-knee amputation into a functional below-knee amputation by using the

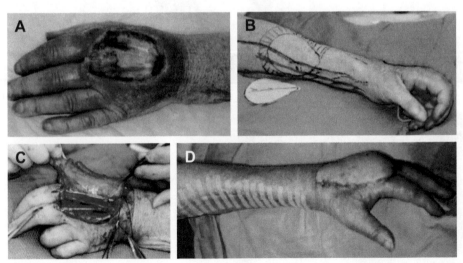

Fig. 3. (*A–D*) Including the palmaris tendon and vascularized fascia as a gliding surface may enhance reconstruction with a radial forearm flap.

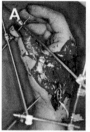
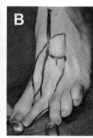
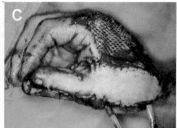
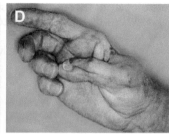

Fig. 4. (*A–D*) Maintaining anything salvageable in this thumb reconstruction allows for the best possible reconstruction.

ankle joint as a pseudo-knee.[18] Functionally, this dramatically reduces energy expenditure and allows placement of a below-knee prosthesis with active knee flexion (**Fig. 5**).

REPLANT WHEN POSSIBLE

Replantation (and now transplantation) offers the ideal use of spare parts and the perfect replacement of like with like. Replantation may be

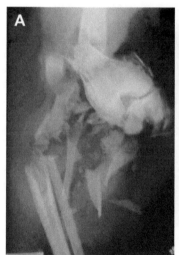
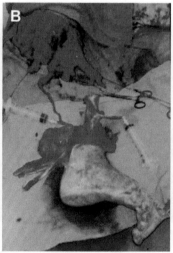
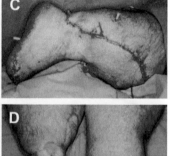
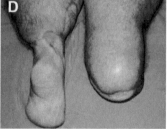

Fig. 5. (*A–E*) Van Nes rotationplasty using the ankle joint as pseudo-knee to convert an above-knee amputation into a functional below-knee amputation.

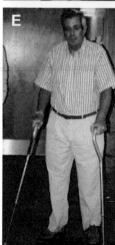

heterotopic or nonanatomic, such as in the hand, where the least traumatized part may be used in the optimal position to maximize function.[17] Even if a part is not salvageable, much can often be saved and used, thereby reducing donor sites.

Sometimes only a portion of the replant survives, but even this can be helpful in reducing

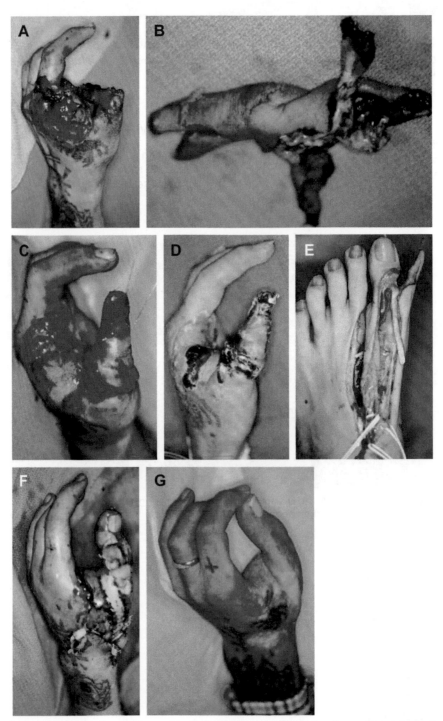

Fig. 6. (A–G) By maintaining what is salvageable form this thumb replant, the donor site morbidity is minimized and the recipient site function is maximized.

donor-site morbidity, as demonstrated in **Fig. 6** where partial salvage of a thumb replant means that only a *soft* tissue from a toe is needed to give an excellent reconstructive result.

Complex wound problems often occur in the head and neck, where highly specialized tissues may be difficult to reconstruct. One example of this is in ear reconstruction whereby revascularizing an ear amputation may be impossible. In this situation, dermabrading the epidermis, reattaching the nonvascularized ear, and burying this beneath a retroauricular pocket to revascularize can allow the part to be saved. Once revascularized, the ear can be partially removed from its pocket and allowed to reepithelialize, attaining an excellent cosmetic result, superior to most multistage reconstructions using heterotopic cartilage (**Fig. 7**).[19]

PRESERVE LENGTH

Preserving the length of extremities and digits during reconstruction and replantation is another core principle when dealing with complex wound problems. One example already mentioned is the use of a Van Nes rotationplasty to convert an otherwise above-knee amputation to a functional below-knee amputation. Similarly in the upper extremity, maintenance of the elbow is important to allow patients to reach their mouth and face for feeding and hygiene.

Segmental injuries provide a unique opportunity for using otherwise untouched distal tissues. In patients requiring resection of a proximal upper extremity or a forequarter amputation, the remaining distal arm may be used to recreate a shoulder girdle. This situation is demonstrated in **Fig. 8**, where an arteriovenous malformation necessitated amputation at the clavicle and humeral level. Using the distal arm as a pedicled flap allows maintenance of a "shoulder girdle." This girdle significantly improves function and allows patients the ability to fit clothes more normally and carry objects such as backpacks, which would otherwise be impossible.

Spare parts from traumatic injuries may also be used to maintain length. A severe train-collision trauma is shown in **Fig. 9**. When multiple extremities are injured, consideration of heterotopic replantation is important. In this case, a fillet of

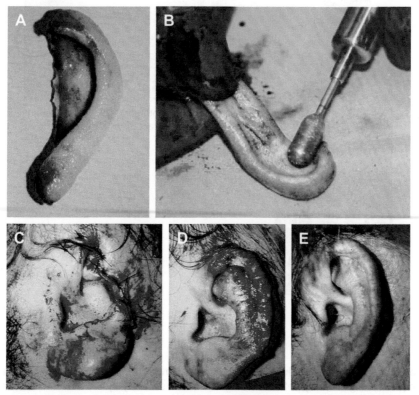

Fig. 7. (*A–E*) An avulsed ear may be de-epithelialized and buried after nonvascularized replantation, and unburied in a delayed fashion to attain an excellent cosmetic result.

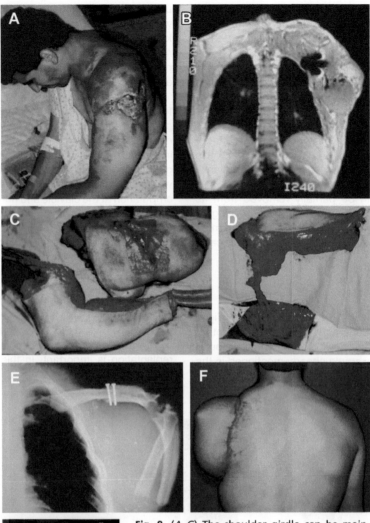

Fig. 8. (*A–G*) The shoulder girdle can be maintained by using an intact distal arm as a pedicled flap, thus allowing a better functional and cosmetic outcome.

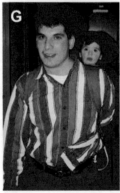

sole was used to resurface a below-knee amputation stump to provide significantly better coverage for the fitting of a prosthesis in the future. The dorsum of the foot and the remaining toes from this lower extremity were heterotopically replanted to the severely injured left hand. Parts of this replantation did not survive, but those parts that did were later rearranged, thereby bringing the great toe into

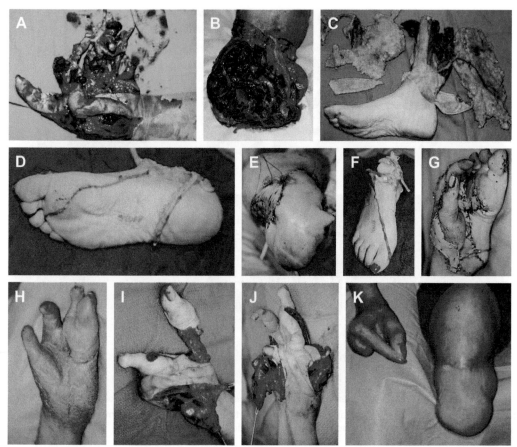

Fig. 9. (*A–K*) When multiple extremities are injured, use of all parts and heterotopic placement may allow length preservation. Here a fillet of the sole is used to create a good load-bearing below-knee amputation surface and the toes are heterotopically replanted to the hand, which after later rearrangement allows for a very functional pinch.

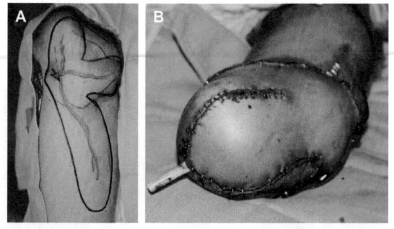

Fig. 10. (*A, B*) Use of a combined scapula and parascapula flap allows durable coverage of a below-knee amputation stump.

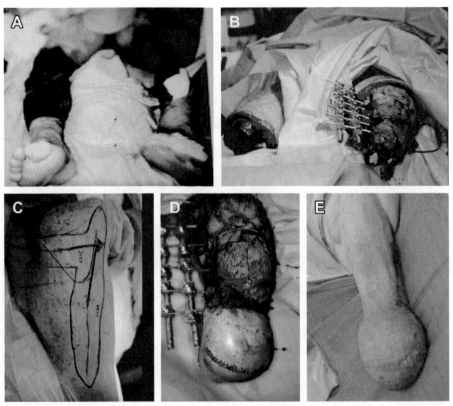

Fig. 11. (*A–E*) Maintaining only the load-bearing surface of this amputation with a combined scapula and parascapula flap maintains length and allows for fitting of a below-knee prosthesis.

a thumb position and again maximizing function while minimizing donor-site morbidity.[20]

Another classic example of maintenance of length is the use of a combined scapula and parascapular flap for coverage of lower extremity wounds. Using a tailored clover-leaf pattern based on the subscapular system, one is able to provide excellent durable soft-tissue coverage over the bony skeleton of

a below-knee amputation, eliminating the need for a higher bony amputation (**Figs. 10** and **11**).

Wounds of the heel may be another complex reconstructive problem. The use of a medial plantar artery flap is an ideal example of using like tissue to reconstruct the heel while skin-grafting the medial plantar surface, which is non–weight-bearing. In this way, any form of amputation is avoided (**Fig. 12**).

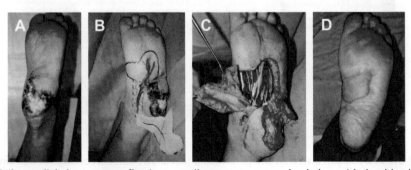

Fig. 12. (*A–D*) The medial plantar artery flap is an excellent way to cover a heel ulcer with durable glabrous tissue.

CONSIDER ALL LAYERS OF TISSUE

Complex wound reconstructions, particularly those of the head and neck, may require attention to be paid to all layers of tissue, and may include reconstructing linings inside flaps such as in the nasal airway.[21] To create a lining, flaps may be used in multiple stages, layered intraoperatively, prelaminated, or multiple flaps may be used to create each layer.[22]

An example of a lining reconstruction is shown in **Fig. 13**. In this patient, nasal collapse has occurred secondary to Wegener granulomatosis. In this case, bilateral facial artery musculomucosal flaps are elevated and brought through the upper buccal sulcus to create adequate lining for nasal reconstruction.[23–25]

In addition, flaps may be harvested in such a way that they already possess lining. One example of this is in the reconstruction of an arteriovenous malformation of the left ala (**Fig. 14**). In this case, a full-thickness nasal ala resection is performed and the ascending auricular helix is used as a free flap to the angular artery. Of note, the configuration of the donor site provides external coverage as well internal lining, producing a very cosmetically acceptable result.[26]

In cases of major reconstruction after very large resections, entire free flaps may need to be used for lining, and the use of multiple free flaps or

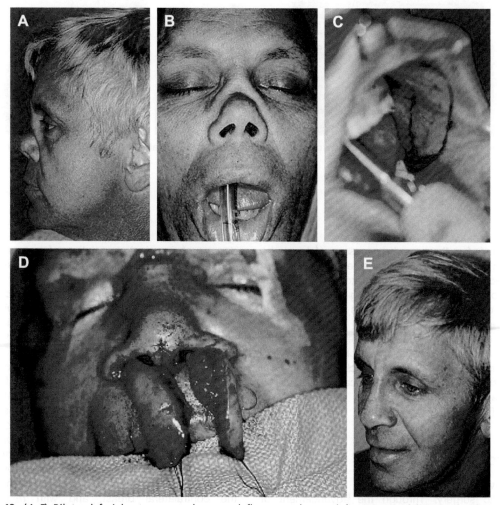

Fig. 13. (*A–E*) Bilateral facial artery musculomucosal flaps may be used for intranasal lining to aid a nasal reconstruction.

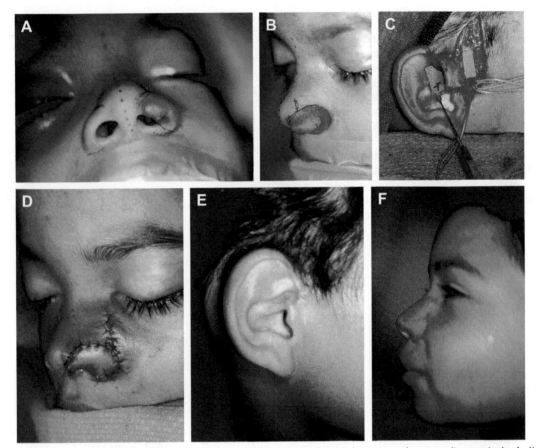

Fig. 14. (*A–F*) Reconstruction of an arteriovenous malformation of the left ala uses the ascending auricular helix with its double-sided skin coverage.

chimeric free flaps may be necessary.[27] As can be seen in **Fig. 15**, a defect after a hemifacial sarcoma resection may be large enough to require a rectus abdominis free flap with overlying skin for lining, followed by an anterolateral thigh flap for external coverage.

In cases where a single-stage operation is not sufficient to provide this lining, prelamination may be used. Complex tissues, such as a full nasal construct, can be "built" in a location such as the forearm, and later elevated as a radial forearm free flap.

INNOVATE

Innovation is essential to the advancement of plastic surgery. Through the advancement of microsurgery and now the use of vascularized composite tissue allotransplantation, an endless

degree of imaginative solutions for countless complex and unique wound problems are possible.

Fig. 16 demonstrates a case of recurrent tibial osteomyelitis. Using a transosseous route for the flap pedicle, a lateral gastrocnemius myocutaneous flap is able to cover the defect and fill in the bony dead space after debridement of the osteomyelitis.[28]

Folded flaps are another innovative way to reconstruct otherwise large and complex defects. The patient shown in **Fig. 17** underwent chest wall resection for dermatofibrosarcoma protuberans as a child. She later underwent a radical excision after sarcoma recurrence. Reconstruction of this defect with a double-pedicled folded transverse rectus abdominis myocutaneous flap provides both the bulk and contour necessary to match the contralateral breast, and with relatively straightforward secondary procedures an excellent cosmetic outcome can be obtained.[29]

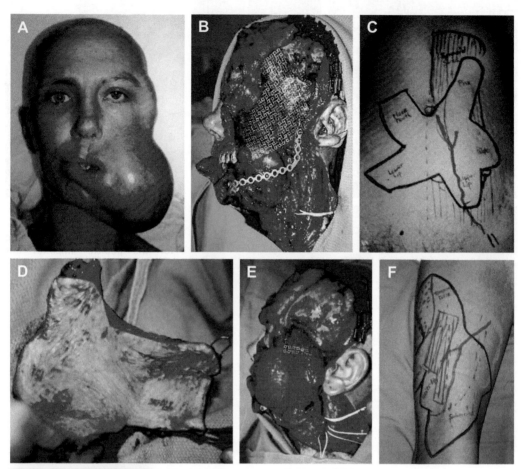

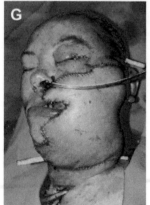

Fig. 15. (A–G) Reconstruction of this hemifacial defect may require multiple free flaps to provide enough tissue as well an internal and external surface.

338

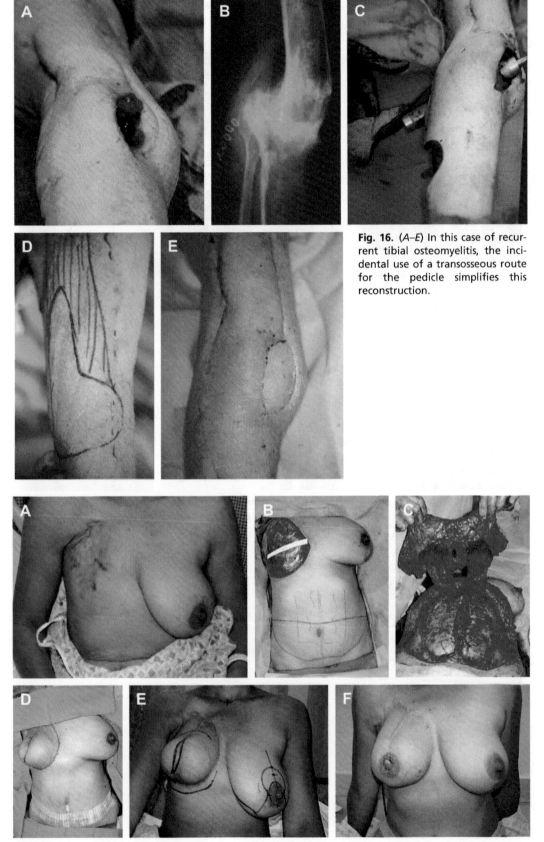

Fig. 16. (*A–E*) In this case of recurrent tibial osteomyelitis, the incidental use of a transosseous route for the pedicle simplifies this reconstruction.

Fig. 17. (*A–F*) Reconstruction of a large chest wall defect with a double-pedicled, folded transverse rectus abdominis myocutaneous flap.

SUMMARY

The approach to complex wound problems in plastic surgery often requires sophisticated surgical options. There is no end of possibilities for reconstruction using the principles of plastic surgery applied to countless wounds that we see as plastic surgeons. Critical to success and outlined herein is a list of things to keep in mind:

1. Planning is critical to the outcome of all plastic surgery procedures, particularly when these are multistage.
2. Keep a lifeboat, as one never knows when a problem will recur or an initial solution will fail.
3. Replace like with like to ensure optimal reconstruction using the best available tissue.
4. Use all spare parts before taking tissue from a virgin donor site.
5. Replant when possible, as amputated parts, whether replaced heterotopically or nonanatomically, are still typically the best reconstructive option.
6. Preserve length whenever possible in reconstructing extremities, to maximize functionality.
7. Consider all tissue layers and, where possible, laminate or fold flaps to obtain lining where this is needed.
8. Innovate when undertaking complex wound reconstruction, as more elegant solutions may be available to those who think laterally.

REFERENCES

1. Taylor GI, Daniel RK. The anatomy of several free flap donor sites. Plast Reconstr Surg 1975;56(3):243–53.
2. Taylor GI, Daniel RK. The free flap: composite tissue transfer by vascular anastomosis. Aust N Z J Surg 1973;43(1):1–3.
3. Pribaz JJ, Maitz PK, Fine NA. Flap prefabrication using the "vascular crane" principle: an experimental study and clinical application. Br J Plast Surg 1994;47(4):250–6.
4. Mathy JA, Pribaz JJ. Prefabrication and prelamination applications in current aesthetic facial reconstruction. Clin Plast Surg 2009;36(3):493–505.
5. Guo L, Pribaz JJ. Clinical flap prefabrication. Plast Reconstr Surg 2009;124(Suppl 6):e340–50.
6. Pribaz JJ, Fine NA. Prelamination: defining the prefabricated flap—a case report and review. Microsurgery 1994;15(9):618–23.
7. Pribaz JJ, Weiss DD, Mulliken JB, et al. Prelaminated free flap reconstruction of complex central facial defects. Plast Reconstr Surg 1999;104(2):357–65 [discussion 366–7].
8. Pribaz JJ, Fine NA. Prefabricated and prelaminated flaps for head and neck reconstruction. Clin Plast Surg 2001;28(2):261–72, vii.
9. D'Arpa S, Cordova A, Pignatti M, et al. Freestyle pedicled perforator flaps: safety, prevention of complications, and management based on 85 consecutive cases. Plast Reconstr Surg 2011;128(4):892–906.
10. Pomahac B, Pribaz J, Eriksson E, et al. Three patients with full facial transplantation. N Engl J Med 2012;366(8):715–22.
11. Pomahac B, Pribaz J, Eriksson E, et al. Restoration of facial form and function after severe disfigurement from burn injury by a composite facial allograft. Am J Transplant 2011;11(2):386–93.
12. Pribaz JJ, Morris DJ, Mulliken JB. Three-dimensional folded free-flap reconstruction of complex facial defects using intraoperative modeling. Plast Reconstr Surg 1994;93(2):285–93.
13. Pribaz JJ, Fine N, Orgill DP. Flap prefabrication in the head and neck: a 10-year experience. Plast Reconstr Surg 1999;103(3):808–20.
14. Russell RC, Neumeister MW, Ostric SA, et al. Extremity reconstruction using nonreplantable tissue ("spare parts"). Clin Plast Surg 2007;34(2):211–22, viii.
15. Pribaz JJ, Morris DJ, Barrall D, et al. Double fillet of foot free flaps for emergency leg and hand coverage with ultimate great toe to thumb transfer. Plast Reconstr Surg 1993;91(6):1151–3.
16. Cavadas PC, Landin L, Thione A. Secondary ectopic transfer for replantation salvage after severe wound infection. Microsurgery 2011;31(4):288–92.
17. Soucacos PN, Beris AE, Malizos KN, et al. Transpositional microsurgery in multiple digital amputations. Microsurgery 1994;15(7):469–73.
18. Krajbich JI, Carroll NC. Van Nes rotationplasty with segmental limb resection. Clin Orthop Relat Res 1990;(256):7–13.
19. Pribaz JJ, Crespo LD, Orgill DP, et al. Ear replantation without microsurgery. Plast Reconstr Surg 1997;99(7):1868–72.
20. Chen HC, O'Brien BM, Pribaz JJ, et al. The use of tonometry in the assessment of upper extremity lymphoedema. Br J Plast Surg 1988;41(4):399–402.
21. Abramson DL, Vander Woude DL, Orgill DP, et al. Traumatic avulsion and reconstruction of the midface. J Craniomaxillofac Trauma 1996;2(1):61–4.
22. Parrett BM, Pribaz JJ. An algorithm for treatment of nasal defects. Clin Plast Surg 2009;36(3):407–20.
23. Pribaz J, Stephens W, Crespo L, et al. A new intraoral flap: facial artery musculomucosal (FAMM) flap. Plast Reconstr Surg 1992;90(3):421–9.
24. Pribaz JJ, Meara JG, Wright S, et al. Lip and vermilion reconstruction with the facial artery musculomucosal flap. Plast Reconstr Surg 2000;105(3):864–72.
25. Duffy FJ Jr, Rossi RM, Pribaz JJ. Reconstruction of Wegener's nasal deformity using bilateral facial artery musculomucosal flaps. Plast Reconstr Surg 1998;101(5):1330–3.

26. Pribaz JJ, Falco N. Nasal reconstruction with auricular microvascular transplant. Ann Plast Surg 1993; 31(4):289–97.

27. Agarwal JP, Agarwal S, Adler N, et al. Refining the intrinsic chimera flap: a review. Ann Plast Surg 2009; 63(4):462–7.

28. Morris DJ, Pribaz JJ. Transtibial transposition of gastrocnemius muscle and musculocutaneous flaps. Br J Plast Surg 1992;45(1):59–61.

29. Chan RK, Pribaz JJ. Refinement in breast reconstruction with folded flaps. Plast Reconstr Surg 2010;126(1):37–9.

An Algorithm for Limb Salvage for Diabetic Foot Ulcers

Joon Pio Hong, MD, PhD, MMM*, Tae Suk Oh, MD

KEYWORDS

- Diabetic foot • Foot ulcers • Limb salvage

KEY POINTS

- A multidisciplinary approach is needed to initially control and treat multiple factors causing severe diabetic foot ulceration.
- Attention should be given to not only the wound but also the whole spectrum of care.
- The surgical steps of debridement, infection control, and vascular intervention are key steps to stabilize the wound and to prepare for a successful reconstruction.
- Reconstruction should provide a well-vascularized tissue to control infection, adequate contour for footwear, durability, and solid anchorage to resist shearing forces during gait.

INTRODUCTION

Chronic ulceration of the lower leg is a frequent condition, with a prevalence of 3% to 5% in the population older than 65 years.[1] The incidence of ulceration is increasing because of the aging population and increased risk factors for atherosclerotic occlusion, such as smoking, obesity, and diabetes. Although most leg ulcers are caused by venous insufficiency (approximately 45%–60%), arterial insufficiency (10%–20%), diabetes (15%–25%), or combinations of these, the most debilitating of them is ulcers caused by diabetes.[2]

According to the statistics given in the United States, approximately 3% to 4% of individuals with diabetes currently have foot ulcers or deep infections and 25% will develop foot ulcers sometime during their life.[3,4] Their risk of lower leg amputation increases by a factor of 8 once an ulcer develops. It is estimated that the age-adjusted rate of lower extremity amputation in patients with diabetes is 15-fold that in individuals without diabetes.[5] Intractable diabetic foot ulcers can bring not only decreased physical, emotional, and social functions but also huge economic impact to the patient.[6–8] Furthermore, the 5-year mortality after major amputations may range from 39% to as high as 80%.[3,9] Hence, salvage for diabetic foot ulcers remains important because it will reduce the economic burden and improve the quality of life.

MULTIDISCIPLINARY APPROACH

The spectrum of diabetic foot disease may vary from asymptomatic to critically ischemic limb with unavoidable amputation. The wide manifestation of symptoms is because of multifactor pathophysiology. The principal pathogenesis involves ischemia, neuropathy, and infection, and the addition of external trauma, peripheral edema, and foot deformity may further increase the risk for diabetic foot ulceration.[10] These conditions may act alone or synergistically to result in Charcot deformities, Achilles tendon contractures, ulcerations, necrosis, and gangrene. One must consider these pathologic conditions and manage them in sequence to provide an efficient care for the foot.

Treatment must begin with strict control of blood glucose level and nutritional support while aggressively managing the wound and infection

Conflict of interest: None to declare.
Department of Plastic Surgery, Asan Medical Center, University of Ulsan College of Medicine, 88 Olympic-ro 43-gil, Songpagu, Seoul 138-736, Korea
* Corresponding author.
E-mail address: joonphong@amc.seoul.kr

Clin Plastic Surg 39 (2012) 341–352
doi:10.1016/j.cps.2012.05.004

to achieve closure of the defect. In patients with ischemic limb, vascular bypass or angioplasty may play a vital role to enhance circulation allowing further reconstruction of soft tissue and bone.

The nurse specialist or coordinator helps to use the team recourses efficiently. After gathering general information about the patient and initial screening of the systemic and foot condition, the specialist would refer to endocrinologist, nutritionist, and proper departments for further treatment and evaluation. There are 4 categories for initial foot evaluation:

1. Vascular
2. Neuropathic
3. Orthopedic
4. Infectious wounds.

Multiple departments may be involved simultaneously to improve the patient's foot condition. In cases of emergent wounds in the authors' center, a plastic surgeon would be notified immediately for emergency debridement and further clinical decision. This is the first and also a major step to limit the spread of acute infection and to salvage of the diabetic foot.[11] The coordinated approach is efficient because no time is wasted waiting for consultations, and it ensures the involvement of proper parties and integrates departments to work closely when undergoing challenging decisions and surgical treatment. **Fig. 1** shows the multidisciplinary algorithm for primary screening and initial treatment of wounds.

With the introduction of a multidisciplinary approach, the trend of management has shifted from major amputation to limb salvage.[12] By addressing the issues of perfusion, infection, wound treatment, off-loading, and bone surgery, the salvage rate is increased. Similar with other reports, the major amputation rate for diabetic foot in the authors' center has reduced significantly after multidisciplinary approach and recently maintains to be about 3% to 4%.[13,14] Although the indications for major amputation still exist and often are caused by multiple factors, such as

- Systemic sepsis
- Major tissue loss
- Significant comorbid factors
- Poor patient compliance
- Nonreconstructable peripheral vascular disease.

the goal remains the same to salvage the limb under good clinical judgment. A nonhealing ulcer itself should not be considered as an indication for amputation but must be explored to solve the underlying pathologic conditions.[15,16]

SPECTRUM OF CARE

When considering diabetic foot for reconstruction, there are multiple issues to be addressed. These issues can be effectively approached through a multidisciplinary approach.

- The first step is to control the systemic aspect of diabetes. Malnutrition, chronic renal disease, and hypertension have to be addressed properly and treatment schedules set before and after surgery, especially hemodialysis and perioperative blood glucose control.
- While the systemic condition of the patient is being optimized, specific attention can be directed to the foot ulcer. Depending on the general condition, peripheral vascular status, bone pathology, wound depth, location, duration, involvement of chronic osteomyelitis, and patient motivation, wounds can be treated with debridement and other related surgical procedures.
- Another important issue is the vascular pathology of the patient. The vascular surgery consultation is essential when the patient is symptomatic with ischemic pain or a nonhealing ulcer. Neuropathic ulcers require debridement of nonviable or infected tissue, combined with local wound care and off-loading.

If the condition of the diabetic wound is not improved by such procedures or aggressive wound care, foot salvage procedures can be considered. A robust predictor of healing is 53% change in the wound area of diabetic foot ulcers.[17] The authors' monitor the change in wound size and depth, and when wound healing is stalled despite good standard of care, such as off-loading, infection control, edema control, and advanced dressings, additional treatment with hyperbaric oxygen, cell therapy, growth factor treatment, and negative pressure wound therapy is considered. Depending on the complexity of the wound, some of these secondary modalities are used primarily as well. The progress of wound healing is closely monitored, and stalled healing, despite these multimodal therapies, may become one of the indicators for reconstruction. **Fig. 2** shows the spectrum of care for diabetic foot ulcers from general care to reconstruction or amputation.

ROLE OF MICROSURGERY

Until recently, reconstruction with microsurgical techniques has been under debate. This was due to the incorrect concept, first attributed to

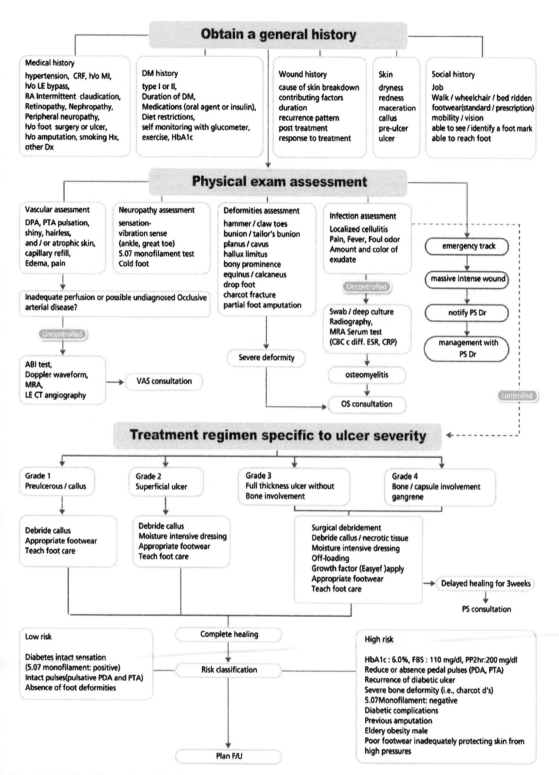

Fig. 1. Multidisciplinary algorithm for primary screening and initial treatment of diabetic foot ulcer. ABI, ankle-brachial index; CBC c diff. ESR, complete blood count with differential erythrocyte sedimentation rate; CRF, chronic renal failure; CRP, C-reactive protein; CT, computed tomography; DM, diabetes mellitus; DPA, diagnostic peritoneal aspiration; LE, lower extremity; MI, myocardial infarction; MRA, magnetic resonance angiography; OS, orthopedic surgery; PDA, patent ductus arteriosus; PS, plastic surgery; PTA, percutaneous transluminal angioplasty; RA, rheumatoid arthritis; VAS, vascular surgery.

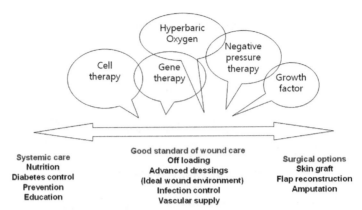

Fig. 2. The wide spectrum of care for diabetic foot ulcers from general/systemic care, good standard of wound care, adjunctive therapies to reconstruction or amputation.

Goldenberg and colleagues[18] in 1959, that patients with diabetes have an increased incidence of small vessel disease that results in foot ulcers. Particularly, it was thought that patients with diabetes have arteriolar occlusive disease, which can cause ischemic lesions. The investigators studied amputation specimens from patients with gangrene and concluded that patients with diabetes have endothelial hypertrophy and proliferation in the smaller arteries, with complete occlusion of the lumen in several cases.

But subsequent studies failed to demonstrate increased arteriolar occlusive disease or endothelial proliferation.[19–21] A thickening of the capillary basement membrane has been documented but not capillary narrowing or occlusion.[19] This same study showed that diabetics often have atherosclerotic occlusion of the tibial arteries, but the occlusive disease occurs mainly in the leg, so that the arterial system in the foot is less involved. Based on these studies, limb salvage from diabetic foot using microsurgical approach showed similar success comparable to that from non-diabetic patients.[22–27] Meta-analysis of a systematic review of free tissue transfer in 528 patients with diabetes in 18 studies showed that flap survival was 92% and limb salvage rate was 83.4% over a 28-month average follow-up period. This study indicates that free tissue transfer in the management of nontraumatic lower extremity wounds in patients with diabetes may avoid amputations.[26] Free flaps and microsurgery technique now play an important role in the salvage of the limb from chronic ulcerations. This review presents a surgical algorithm for limb salvage focused on the microsurgical reconstruction (**Fig. 3**).

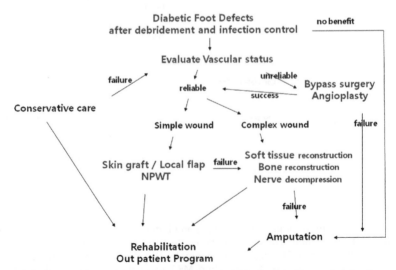

Fig. 3. Surgical algorithm for limb salvage. Important steps include debridement, infection control, vascular status evaluation with intervention, and reconstruction.

Pearls and pitfalls

The use of this algorithm gives one a general guideline on important steps:

Pearls

1. Good standard of care, including debridement, dressing, off-loading, and edema control
2. Vascular intervention
3. Reconstruction with local and free flaps

Pitfalls

One must understand that this is not an absolute step-by-step approach but rather a back and forth approach. Decision for amputation should not be made easily and all efforts should be taken, including exploration for recipient vessels, to ensure that there is no alternative to amputation.

SURGICAL ALGORITHM

- Although the medical care for the patient with diabetic foot ulceration begins with stabilization of the patient, the surgical care begins with debridement and control of infection.
- After the patient and the wound are stabilized, further evaluation of the wound is made.
- Unless indicated for major amputation, the reconstructive algorithm is followed.
- If the wound is simple with minimal or no vital structures exposed, conservative care with various treatments can be considered.
- If the wound is well granulating after wound preparation, skin graft or a small local flap can be performed.[28] A well-granulating wound itself is an indication for good vascularity.
- If healing is stalling, then further evaluation using transcutaneous oxygen pressure measurement (TcPo$_2$) or angiograms may be necessary to evaluate the arterial flow and prepare for vascular intervention.
- The same evaluation and approach to ensure vascularity are needed for complex wounds waiting reconstructive procedure.

DEBRIDEMENT

The initial steps in the treatment of diabetic foot wound are to[29]

1. Evaluate
2. Debride
3. Treat infection

Lack of timely management will lead to amputations and longer hospital stays.[30] Optimal management of diabetic foot infection can reduce incidence of major limb amputations and other related morbidities.

- If symptoms and sign of infection are clinically suspected, proper treatment must be provided without delay.
- If superficial infection is suspected, without systemic infection, antibiotic treatment along with nonweight bearing of the foot should ensue.
- All nonviable and infected soft tissue and bone should be excised during debridement. Milking along the proximal tendon can be helpful to identify and limit the ascending infection. Tissue culture should be sent.
- Sufficient irrigation should follow debridement to reduce bacterial count.[31]
- Recent advances in technology introduce a hydrosurgery system that allows one to debride and irrigate simultaneously, while preserving viable tissues, allowing reduced surgical time.[32,33]

The understanding of vascular distribution of the foot, angiosome, helps to plan not only reconstruction but also debridement (**Fig. 4**).[34] When planning for reconstruction, one should design a local flap by not violating the angiosome territory, which may lead to flap breakdown (**Fig. 5**).[35] Also, by performing debridement guided by the angiosome territory, flap survival is enhanced by increasing the chance for marginal vascularization from healthy surrounding angiosome territory.

Repetitive debridement should be performed as part of wound preparation for reconstruction while monitoring C-reactive protein for possible hidden infections and using it as an index for possible infection after reconstruction.

VASCULAR INTERVENTION

In the author's surgical algorithm, all patients considered for microsurgical reconstruction undergo a noninvasive computed tomography (CT)-angiogram to evaluate the vascular status. The CT-angiogram provides information regarding general vascular anatomy of the lower extremity and shows artherosclerotic change of vessels, which is useful when choosing recipient vessels.

CT-Angiogram

The overview is important because collateral vessels may be the main trunk to the distal limb

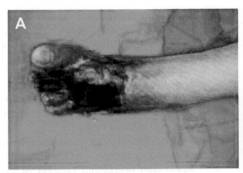
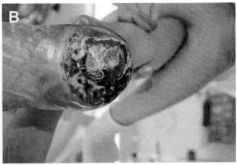

Fig. 4. Skin necrosis over the angiosome of dorsalis pedis. Note how the defect correlates to the angiosome (*A*). Necrosis of the heel is noted in correlation with calcaneal branch of peroneal artery (*B*).

(**Fig. 6**). Without this information, one may elevate the flap harvesting the main arterial source to the distal limb, causing limb ischemia. If vascular status is in doubt, then revascularization by angioplasty or bypass surgery is referred. Although preoperative angiograms may indicate intact anatomy of the artery to the foot, actual findings on surgery can be different.

Ultrasound Duplex Scans

To confirm the distal vascular flow, we use ultrasound duplex scans.

A study by Kim and Lee[36] showed correlation of peak blood flow velocity of more than 40 cm/s to flap survival. However, in an ongoing study at our center, the authors hypothesized that the preoperative measurement of flow will not influence the

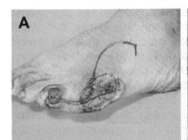
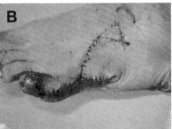
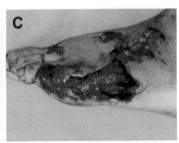

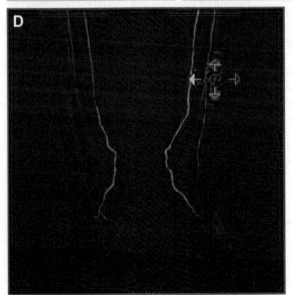

Fig. 5. Poor design violating the angiosome concept leading to local flap breakdown (*A–C*). The follow-up computed tomography- angiogram revealed poor vascular supply of the dorsalis pedis providing insight for breakdown (*D*). *Arrows*, navigation cursor for PACS (picture archives communication system).

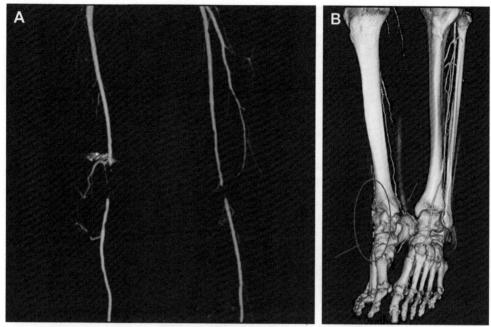

Fig. 6. The need for CT-angiogram is shown, as the descending branch of the circumflex femoral artery is the main collateral of the distal perfusion of the limb. If one were to harvest anterolateral thigh perforator flap then a catastrophic loss of the entire limb may be possible (*A*). The CT-angiogram also provides good information on where the recipient vessel segment is spared from atherosclerosis. The anterior tibial and dorsalis pedis arteries are barely seen (*circled*), whereas the posterior tibial artery is well presented (*right arrow*) (*B*).

survival of the flap, but the perioperative flow will play a more important factor. For now, ultrasound duplex scan provides information in the selection of recipient vessels or to refer for vascular intervention when no recipient vessels can be identified.

TcPo2

The TcPo2 also plays a role in the authors' protocol. Measurement of greater than 30 mm Hg in normobaric oxygen is a relative predictive factor for successful healing, whereas pressure less than that of 30 mm Hg is likely to follow an unfavorable course.[37,38] The wound, if measured under this level after vascular intervention, was treated with hyperbaric oxygen. If peri-wound TcPo2 was greater than 30 mm Hg then further treatment including reconstructive procedures were planned, otherwise amputations at according levels were performed.

Perfusion

The ankle-brachial index (ABI) is not used because it is not reliable in patients with diabetes because of the high incidence of calcified vessels, causing falsely elevated values.[39] In patients with diabetes, the most significant atherosclerosis occlusions occur in the crural arteries, often sparing the arteries of the foot.[19] Bypass to dorsalis pedis or posterior

tibial artery of the foot or angioplasty with or without stent placement procedures result in high success to restore perfusion pressure to the distal circulation of the foot, reestablishing palpable pulse.

Timing of Reconstruction

The timing of reconstruction after vascular intervention is not clear. Reports have shown successful free flap transfer with simultaneous vascular reconstruction to salvage the limb.[40] But early bypass failures within 30 days are reported to be high.[25,41] In the authors' experience, partial flap loss or total loss was suddenly noted after 2 to 3 weeks in patients who underwent vascular intervention with simultaneous reconstruction or reconstruction following few days after vascular interventions, which may suggest that there should be a sufficient stabilization period after vascular intervention.

Reperfusion is most essential before microsurgery reconstruction. If vascular intervention fails and wound progresses, amputation is warranted.

SOFT TISSUE RECONSTRUCTION

Once an adequate debridement and reasonable vascular perfusion is achieved, in extensive and complex diabetic foot defects, reconstruction should be considered. In the author's experience,

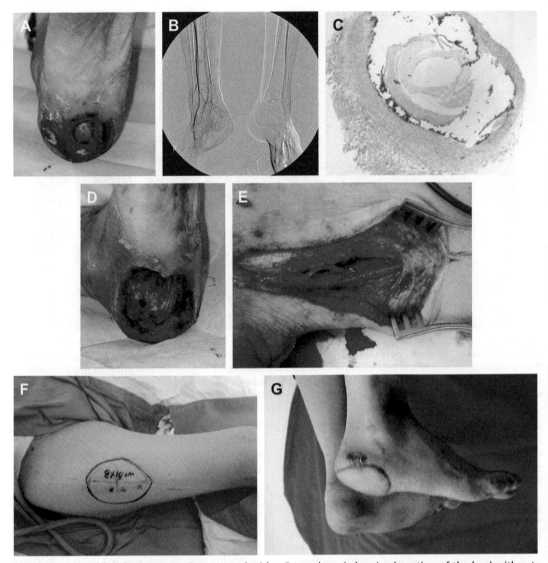

Fig. 7. A 42-year-old diabetic woman is presented with a 3-year long ischemic ulceration of the heel with osteomyelitis (*A*). Angiogram revealed barely patent posterior tibial artery (*B*). The histology of the artery confirms the atherosclerosis (*C*). Complete debridement was performed including the bone (*D*). Recipient artery was explored and posterior tibial artery showed a good pulse while having a short segment spared from calcification (*E*). The anterolateral thigh flap was elevated and artery anastomosed in end to side manner (*F*). The follow-up at 18 months shows good contour without recurrence of osteomyelitis and ulceration (*G*).

local flaps, such as reverse sural, medial plantar, or lateral supramalleolar flaps for large defects, have not been as successful as free flap reconstruction. When reconstructing diabetic foot with reduced vascular flow, the use of local flaps may breach the distal flow of the small collateral vessels. Current vascular status and future flow in which small collateral vessels may play an important role for distal circulation must be considered. Hence, the author's choice for moderate and large defects is the reconstructive microsurgery to transfer free flaps. An inclusion

criteria from a meta-analysis of free tissue transfer in 528 patients with diabetes in 18 studies suggests

1. Lower limb defect, which has not displayed any signs of granulation or healing despite adequate debridement or necrotic tissue and conservative treatment
2. No significant renal function impairment
3. No significant systemic illness likely to be exacerbated by multiple operations and prolong rehabilitation

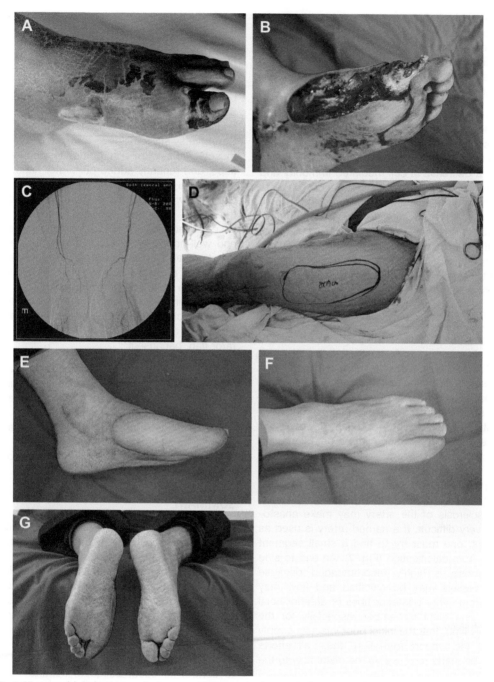

Fig. 8. A 65-year-old diabetic man is shown with ischemic change, infection, and osteomyelitis of the first ray of the foot (*A*). Complete debridement is performed according to the angiosome concept while sparing the first phalangeal bone (*B*). The angiogram of the patient showed poor supply of dorsalis pedis as suspected and a branch of the posterior tibial artery was identified (*C*). A thin anterolateral thigh flap with dimension of 8 × 17 cm was raised, pedicles anastomosed and the flap wrapped around the defect (*D*). Follow-up at 18 months shows good contour of the foot without recurrence of osteomyelitis and recurrence of ulceration (*E–G*).

4. Previously ambulatory with the aim to restore a functional limb
5. Likely to engage with the significant physiotherapy required for return to normal living
6. Peak flow velocity of greater than 40 cm/s in recipient artery.

The authors generally agree with the suggested inclusion criteria except for the significant renal disease. In their experience, they have not found an increased risk for failure despite uremia may cause a decrease in cell-mediated immunity and impair wound healing.[42,43] However, patients after kidney transplantation had an odds ratio of 4.857 of having flap failure ($P = .041$). The author prefers to present the contraindication rather than the indications for flap reconstruction as microsurgery technique evolves using small recipient vessels rather than major vessels for reconstruction.[44]

Recipient Vessel

The most important factor may be the perfusion of the recipient vessel. A small vessel with good pulsatile flow is indicated for microsurgery. Thus an absolute contraindication would be no flow to the foot without any sign of perfusion from any distal small vessels. This supermicrosurgery and free style reconstruction approach, however, will require a refined skill along with a paradigm shift for reconstruction.

The biggest challenge in reconstructive microsurgery for diabetic foot is finding the recipient vessel. Even with an adequate flow to the foot, atherosclerosis of the artery may make anastomosis very difficult. If a named artery is used as recipient, one must try to find a small segment spared from calcification (**Fig. 7**). An end to side anastomosis is highly recommended because major vessels may be calcified and flow may come from either posterior tibial or anterior tibial artery. One must remember, especially for the ischemic limb, that the initial poor vascular supply caused the wound formation, thus, all efforts should be made to preserve the distal flow to the foot.

There also has been a report of steal phenomenon in which flow may be diverted to low resistance vascular bed of the new flap.[45,46] In my experience, using the branch from the major artery as a recipient may be a better choice. Rarely branches from posterior tibial and dorsalis pedis arteries are calcified, and by using this branch, one can easily anastomose to a supple and soft artery without diminishing distal flow. An alternative anastomosis may be the T-style anastomosis in which the bypassing artery segment with a branch to the flap is inter-anastomosed between the proximal and distal recipient artery.

Flaps

The flap for reconstruction of diabetic foot should provide a well-vascularized tissue to control infection, adequate contour for footwear, durability, and solid anchorage to resist shearing forces. Controversy still remains as to which flap, whether muscle flaps with skin grafts, fasciocutaneous flaps, and recently added perforator flaps, offers the optimal solution to reconstruct the foot, especially the weight-bearing surface. But as long as the large defect is covered with any well-vascularized tissue, it will provide an independent and well-nourished vascular supply to eradicate infection and increase local oxygen tension, enhancing antibiotic activity and neovascularization to the adjacent ischemic tissue.[47,48] In the author's clinical experience there is a shift toward using perforator flaps, such as anterolateral thigh perforator and superficial circumflex iliac perforator flap, because it[23]

- Provides a thin flap to minimize shearing
- Can take only the superficial fat to imitate the fibrous septa of the sole to adhere tightly
- Enhances neovascularization of the subdermal plexus with adjacent tissue
- Provides adequate blood supply to fight infection (**Fig. 8**).

SUMMARY

In the authors' recent review of diabetic foot reconstruction with free flaps of 171 cases with this algorithm showed flap survival of 91.7%. A multidisciplinary approach is needed to initially control and treat multiple factors causing severe diabetic foot ulceration. The surgical steps of debridement, infection control, and vascular intervention are key steps to stabilize the wound and to prepare for a successful reconstruction. Reconstruction should provide a well-vascularized tissue to control infection, adequate contour for footwear, durability, and solid anchorage to resist shearing forces during gait. Rehabilitation after reconstruction should address the issue of adequate footwear and gait. Education must be provided to teach how to manage and care one's feet. Regular follow-up at the clinic should be made to ensure new changes in life are enforced to prevent repetitive ulceration. This algorithm describes the key factors and steps to increase the chance for successful reconstruction, which will lead to better quality of life and survival.

Summary of first-person experience

The reconstruction of a diabetic foot remains a challenge. In most limbs lost with diabetes, the main causes are infection and ischemia. Time factor plays a major role, and one must be ready to start the treatment of severe infections and ischemia. This is a very difficult task, and in my experience, passion and dedication from the surgeons are required to manage this task. Never give up easily on any limb with chronic ulcers and try to find the cause and improve the pathologic condition. Share the pain of the patients and empathize with them in making difficult decisions like amputations. Give them hope as even after amputations you will have to see them for the rest of their lives. Begin surgical reconstruction with relatively easier cases such as neuropathic types and build your skills toward ischemic one. I really encourage all plastic surgeons to take on this difficult task because treating diabetic ulceration is rewarding and life saving.

REFERENCES

1. Mekkes JR, Loots MA, Van Der Wal AC, et al. Causes, investigation and treatment of leg ulceration. Br J Dermatol 2003;148(3):388–401.
2. Lipsky BA, Berendt AR, Deery HG, et al. Diagnosis and treatment of diabetic foot infections. Plast Reconstr Surg 2006;117(Suppl 7):212S–38S.
3. Reiber GE. The epidemiology of diabetic foot problems. Diabet Med 1996;13(Suppl 1):S6–11.
4. Singh N, Armstrong DG, Lipsky BA. Preventing foot ulcers in patients with diabetes. JAMA 2005;293(2):217–28.
5. Most RS, Sinnock P. The epidemiology of lower extremity amputations in diabetic individuals. Diabetes Care 1983;6(1):87–91.
6. Saar WE, Lee TH, Berlet GC. The economic burden of diabetic foot and ankle disorders. Foot Ankle Int 2005;26(1):27–31.
7. Apelqvist J, Ragnarson-Tennvall G, Larsson J, et al. Long-term costs for foot ulcers in diabetic patients in a multidisciplinary setting. Foot Ankle Int 1995;16(7):388–94.
8. Reiber GE, Lipsky BA, Gibbons GW. The burden of diabetic foot ulcers. Am J Surg 1998;176(Suppl 2A):5S–10S.
9. Moulik PK, Mtonga R, Gill GV. Amputation and mortality in new-onset diabetic foot ulcers stratified by etiology. Diabetes Care 2003;26(2):491–4.
10. Boulton AJ. The diabetic foot: from art to science. The 18th Camillo Golgi lecture. Diabetologia 2004;47(8):1343–53.
11. Childers BJ, Potyondy LD, Nachreiner R, et al. Necrotizing fasciitis: a fourteen-year retrospective study of 163 consecutive patients. Am Surg 2002;68(2):109–16.
12. Wraight PR, Lawrence SM, Campbell DA, et al. Creation of a multidisciplinary, evidence based, clinical guideline for the assessment, investigation and management of acute diabetes related foot complications. Diabet Med 2005;22(2):127–36.
13. Krishnan N, Becker DF. Characterization of a bifunctional PutA homologue from Bradyrhizobium japonicum and identification of an active site residue that modulates proline reduction of the flavin adenine dinucleotide cofactor. Biochemistry 2005;44(25):9130–9.
14. Holstein P, Ellitsgaard N, Olsen BB, et al. Decreasing incidence of major amputations in people with diabetes. Diabetologia 2000;43(7):844–7.
15. Apelqvist J. Wound healing in diabetes. Outcome and costs. Clin Podiatr Med Surg 1998;15(1):21–39.
16. Cavanagh PR, Ulbrecht JS, Caputo GM. The nonhealing diabetic foot wound: fact or fiction? Ostomy Wound Manage 1998;44(Suppl 3A):6S–12S [discussion: 13S].
17. Sheehan P, Jones P, Giurini JM, et al. Percent change in wound area of diabetic foot ulcers over a 4-week period is a robust predictor of complete healing in a 12-week prospective trial. Plast Reconstr Surg 2006;117(Suppl 7):239S–44S.
18. Goldenberg S, Alex M, Joshi RA, et al. Nonatheromatous peripheral vascular disease of the lower extremity in diabetes mellitus. Diabetes 1959;8(4):261–73.
19. Strandness DE Jr, Priest RE, Gibbons GE. Combined clinical and pathologic study of diabetic and nondiabetic peripheral arterial disease. Diabetes 1964;13:366–72.
20. Conrad MC. Large and small artery occlusion in diabetics and nondiabetics with severe vascular disease. Circulation 1967;36(1):83–91.
21. LoGerfo FW, Coffman JD. Current concepts. Vascular and microvascular disease of the foot in diabetes. Implications for foot care. N Engl J Med 1984;311(25):1615–9.
22. Colen LB. Limb salvage in the patient with severe peripheral vascular disease: the role of microsurgical free-tissue transfer. Plast Reconstr Surg 1987;79(3):389–95.
23. Hong JP. Reconstruction of the diabetic foot using the anterolateral thigh perforator flap. Plast Reconstr Surg 2006;117(5):1599–608.
24. Searles JM Jr, Colen LB. Foot reconstruction in diabetes mellitus and peripheral vascular insufficiency. Clin Plast Surg 1991;18(3):467–83.
25. Shenaq SM, Dinh TA. Foot salvage in arteriolosclerotic and diabetic patients by free flaps after vascular bypass: report of two cases. Microsurgery 1989;10(4):310–4.

26. Fitzgerald O'Connor EJ, Vesely M, Holt PJ, et al. A systematic review of free tissue transfer in the management of non-traumatic lower extremity wounds in patients with diabetes. Eur J Vasc Endovasc Surg 2011;41(3):391–9.

27. Oishi SN, Levin LS, Pederson WC. Microsurgical management of extremity wounds in diabetics with peripheral vascular disease. Plast Reconstr Surg 1993;92(3):485–92.

28. Knox KR, Datiashvili RO, Granick MS. Surgical wound bed preparation of chronic and acute wounds. Clin Plast Surg 2007;34(4):633–41.

29. Attinger CE, Bulan EJ. Debridement. The key initial first step in wound healing. Foot Ankle Clin 2001; 6(4):627–60.

30. Reiber GE, Vileikyte L, Boyko EJ, et al. Causal pathways for incident lower-extremity ulcers in patients with diabetes from two settings. Diabetes Care 1999;22(1):157–62.

31. Badia JM, Torres JM, Tur C, et al. Saline wound irrigation reduces the postoperative infection rate in guinea pigs. J Surg Res 1996;63(2):457–9.

32. Granick M, Boykin J, Gamelli R, et al. Toward a common language: surgical wound bed preparation and debridement. Wound Repair Regen 2006; 14(Suppl 1):S1–10.

33. Granick MS, Posnett J, Jacoby M, et al. Efficacy and cost-effectiveness of a high-powered parallel waterjet for wound debridement. Wound Repair Regen 2006;14(4):394–7.

34. Clemens MW, Attinger CE. Angiosomes and wound care in the diabetic foot. Foot Ankle Clin 2010;15(3): 439–64.

35. Attinger C, Cooper P, Blume P, et al. The safest surgical incisions and amputations applying the angiosome principles and using the Doppler to assess the arterial-arterial connections of the foot and ankle. Foot Ankle Clin 2001;6(4):745–99.

36. Kim JY, Lee YJ. A study of the survival factors of free flap in older diabetic patients. J Reconstr Microsurg 2007;23(7):373–80.

37. Christensen KS, Klarke M. Transcutaneous oxygen measurement in peripheral occlusive disease. An indicator of wound healing in leg amputation. J Bone Joint Surg Br 1986;68(3):423–6.

38. Got I. Transcutaneous oxygen pressure (TcPo2): advantages and limitations. Diabetes Metab 1998; 24(4):379–84 [in French].

39. Goss DE, de Trafford J, Roberts VC, et al. Raised ankle/brachial pressure index in insulin-treated diabetic patients. Diabet Med 1989;6(7):576–8.

40. Randon C, Jacobs B, De Ryck F, et al. 15-year experience with combined vascular reconstruction and free flap transfer for limb-salvage. Eur J Vasc Endovasc Surg 2009;38(3):338–45.

41. Bush HL Jr, Nabseth DC, Curl GR, et al. In situ saphenous vein bypass grafts for limb salvage. A current fad or a viable alternative to reversed vein bypass grafts? Am J Surg 1985;149(4):477–80.

42. Yue DK, McLennan S, Marsh M, et al. Effects of experimental diabetes, uremia, and malnutrition on wound healing. Diabetes 1987;36(3):295–9.

43. Berman SJ. Infections in patients with end-stage renal disease. An overview. Infect Dis Clin North Am 2001;15(3):709–20, vii.

44. Hong JP. The use of supermicrosurgery in lower extremity reconstruction: the next step in evolution. Plast Reconstr Surg 2009;123(1):230–5.

45. Rainer C, Schwabegger AH, Meirer R, et al. Microsurgical management of the diabetic foot. J Reconstr Microsurg 2003;19(8):543–53.

46. Sonntag BV, Murphy RX Jr, Chernofsky MA, et al. Microvascular steal phenomenon in lower extremity reconstruction. Ann Plast Surg 1995;34(3):336–9 [discussion: 9–40].

47. Shestak KC, Hendricks DL, Webster MW. Indirect revascularization of the lower extremity by means of microvascular free-muscle flap–a preliminary report. J Vasc Surg 1990;12(5):581–5.

48. Chang N, Mathes SJ. Comparison of the effect of bacterial inoculation in musculocutaneous and random-pattern flaps. Plast Reconstr Surg 1982;70(1):1–10.

Index

Moving?

Make sure your subscription moves with you!

To notify us of your new address, find your **Clinics Account Number** (located on your mailing label above your name), and contact customer service at:

Email: journalscustomerservice-usa@elsevier.com

800-654-2452 (subscribers in the U.S. & Canada)
314-447-8871 (subscribers outside of the U.S. & Canada)

Fax number: 314-447-8029

Elsevier Health Sciences Division
Subscription Customer Service
3251 Riverport Lane
Maryland Heights, MO 63043

*To ensure uninterrupted delivery of your subscription, please notify us at least 4 weeks in advance of move.

ELSEVIER

Printed and bound by CPI Group (UK) Ltd, Croydon, CR0 4YY

03/10/2024

01040355-0008